The Asian Flu
Pandemic of 1957

Stephanie Lundquist-Arora

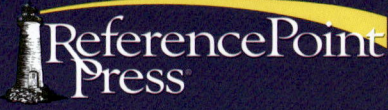

ReferencePoint
Press®

San Diego, CA

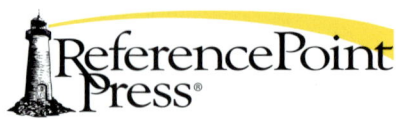
ReferencePoint
Press®

About the Author

Stephanie Lundquist-Arora has master's degrees in political science and public administration. She experienced a pandemic firsthand in July 2009 when she fell ill with the swine flu in Australia. When not writing, Lundquist-Arora likes traveling with her husband and three sons, jogging, reading, painting, learning jiu jitsu, and trying new foods.

© 2022 ReferencePoint Press, Inc.
Printed in the United States

For more information, contact:
ReferencePoint Press, Inc.
PO Box 27779
San Diego, CA 92198
www.ReferencePointPress.com

LIBRARY OF CONGRESS CATALOGING-IN-PUBLICATION DATA

Names: Lundquist-Arora, Stephanie, author.
Title: The Asian flu pandemic of 1957 / Stephanie Lundquist-Arora.
Description: San Diego, CA : ReferencePoint Press, 2022. | Series: Historic
  pandemics and plagues | Includes bibliographical references and index.
Identifiers: LCCN 2020056768 (print) | LCCN 2020056769 (ebook) | ISBN
  9781678200961 (library binding) | ISBN 9781678200978 (ebook other)
Subjects: LCSH: Influenza--History--20th century--Juvenile literature. |
  Epidemics--History--20th century. | Asian flu--Juvenile literature. |
  Epidemics--History--20th century.
Classification: LCC RC150.4 .L86 2022 (print) | LCC RC150.4 (ebook) | DDC
  614.5/18--dc23
LC record available at https://lccn.loc.gov/2020056768
LC ebook record available at https://lccn.loc.gov/2020056769

CONTENTS

Important Events During the Asian Flu Pandemic

1956
The first case of Asian flu is reported in the Guizhou province of southwestern China.

June 1957
On June 2 the pandemic reaches western Europe when an infected person travels on an airplane from Jakarta, Indonesia, to the Netherlands.

April 1957
Predicting that the virus would become a pandemic, Maurice Hilleman, chief of the Department of Respiratory Diseases at Walter Reed Army Medical Center, sends a cable to an army medical general laboratory in Zama, Japan, requesting virus samples.

February 1957
The Asian flu is reported in Singapore.

June 1957
On June 2 some of the first cases of Asian flu are reported in the United States among the crews of several destroyers (warships) at Newport Naval Station in Rhode Island.

1956 / 1957

May 1957
On May 17 Hilleman receives a virus sample from an ill member of the US Navy who had been to Hong Kong. He then sends virus samples to pharmaceutical companies and encourages them to quickly develop a vaccine.

June 1957
Over 1 million cases of the Asian flu are reported throughout India. In Japan, an estimated 70,000 children are afflicted with the flu, and eighty-seven schools close in response.

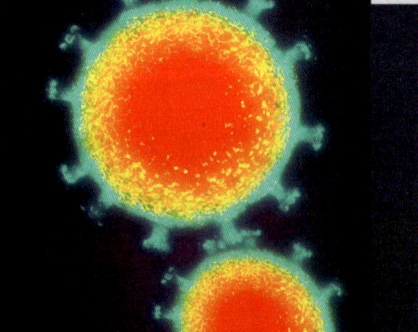

May 1957
On May 21 the SS *Rajula*, a large passenger and cargo ship carrying 1,622 travelers and 200 crew members, docks at the port of Madras on the southeastern coast of India. Many aboard the ship, which had sailed from Singapore, are already suffering from the Asian flu.

June 1957

On June 7 the World Health Organization refers to the Asian flu as a mild epidemic of influenza.

June 1957

On June 29 a high school student from California travels to Grinnell, Iowa, to attend a Presbyterian youth meeting at Grinnell College. She develops symptoms on her way there and exposes 1,680 delegates from over forty states and ten other countries to the virus.

July 1957

Starting on July 11, Valley Forge, Pennsylvania, hosts the weeklong International Boy Scout Jamboree, with fifty-three thousand participants, including Scouts and leaders, from every state and several countries. From the beginning of the event, attendees from California, Louisiana, and Puerto Rico have exhibited symptoms of what turns out to be the Asian flu, which quickly spreads to other attendees.

August 1957

After repeatedly refusing to be vaccinated, US president Dwight Eisenhower gets his Asian flu vaccination on August 26.

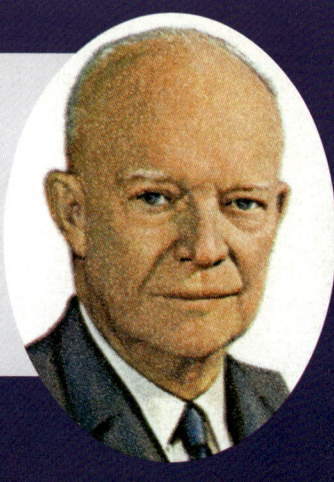

1957   / **1968**

June 1957

On June 23 the pharmaceutical corporation Merck & Co. announces that it has created an Asian flu vaccine that it can mass-produce.

July 1957

The pandemic reaches Saudi Arabia, Kuwait, Yemen, Syria, Iran, Iraq, and Jordan, often by way of foreign traders and pilgrims to Mecca.

1968

Public health officials announce that the Asian flu virus is extinct in the human population.

October 1957

The United States experiences the peak of the pandemic. Some schools close, and others record absenteeism rates of 30 percent.

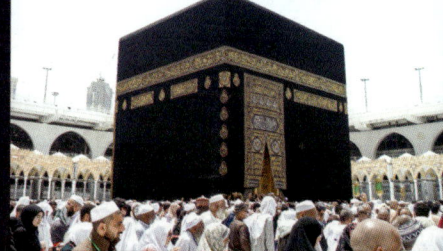

September 1957

Manufacturers produce 40 million doses of the vaccine.

A Quick Response Saves Lives

When Maurice Hilleman, an American microbiologist, took a position with Walter Reed Army Medical Center in 1948, his job was to prevent the next influenza pandemic. For nearly a decade afterward, he bided his time, learning all he could about influenza. In April 1957, when he read an article in the newspaper detailing the influenza situation in Hong Kong, he knew right away that the world was facing a pandemic. Many researchers have subsequently agreed that Hilleman was the right man for the job of fighting the pandemic of 1957 and credit him for its demise. In 2020 *Scientific American* wrote this praise: "Pioneering virologist Maurice Hilleman . . . detected that pandemic from across the globe, convinced reluctant U.S. health officials to take notice, and single-handedly fostered a vaccine that became publicly available. All in just four months."[1]

A Virus Becomes a Pandemic

The new influenza virus had first revealed itself in Guizhou, China, in 1956, and then appeared in Singapore in February 1957 before reaching Hong Kong and spreading quickly from there. Having originated in East Asia, the new strain of influenza widely became known in the media and among public health officials as the "Asian flu."

After spreading across East Asia, the virus reached India in June 1957. By the end of that month, the densely populated country was contending with over 1 million cases of the novel influenza virus. Throughout the summer, the virus touched every other continent, brought by travelers, military personnel, and traders. During the months that followed, the world was faced with the second-worst influenza pandemic of the twentieth century. Whereas the 1918 Spanish flu pandemic, which never witnessed a vaccine, killed an estimated 50 million people worldwide, the Asian flu took an estimated 1.1 million to 2 million lives before a vaccine limited its lethality.

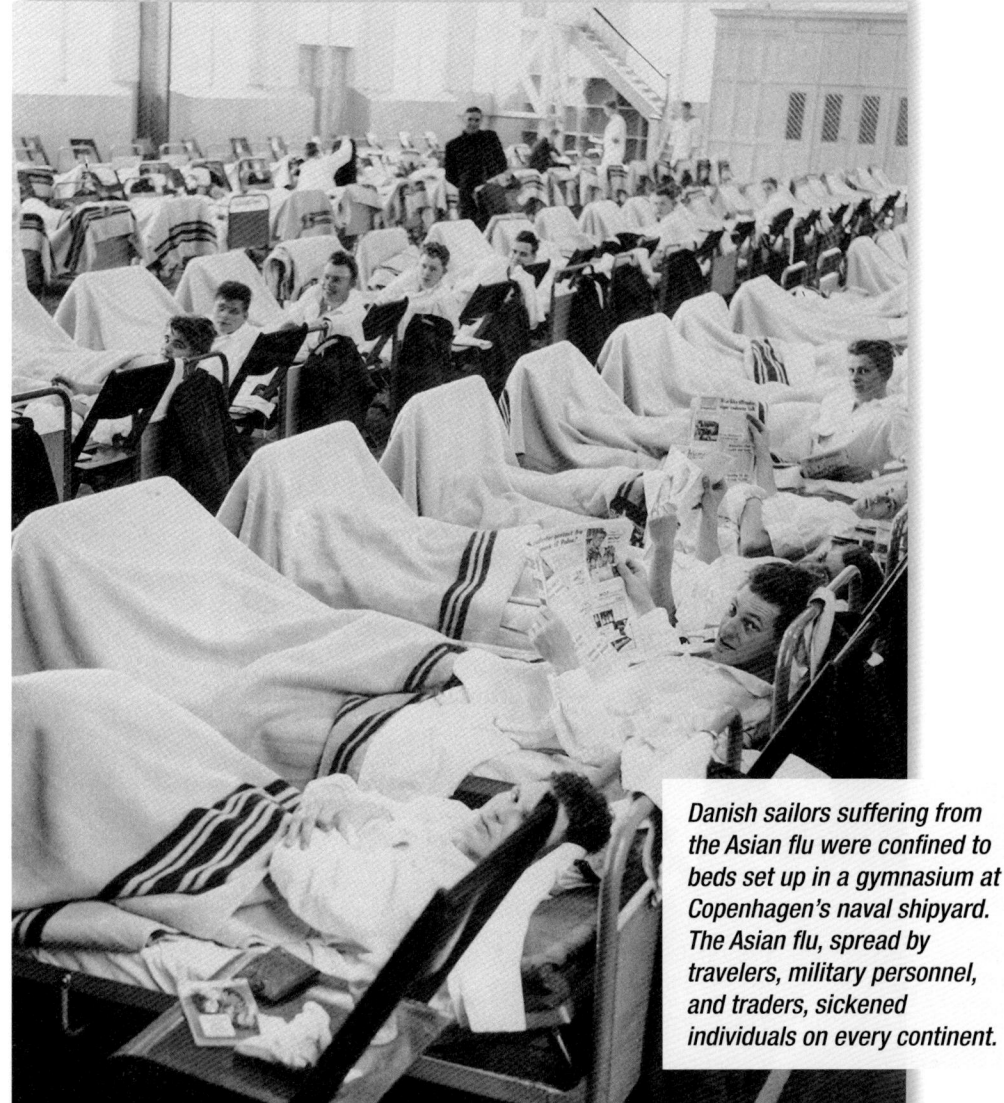

Danish sailors suffering from the Asian flu were confined to beds set up in a gymnasium at Copenhagen's naval shipyard. The Asian flu, spread by travelers, military personnel, and traders, sickened individuals on every continent.

Hilleman understood the severity of the impending pandemic, but other public health experts and doctors disagreed about the significance of the Asian flu. Although they concurred that the Asian flu was highly contagious and many people would become afflicted, not all believed its consequences would be catastrophic. Complications from the virus, including pneumonia and bronchitis, tended to most affect those under age five and over sixty-five, as well as pregnant women. Most of the deaths from the Asian flu were the result of pneumonia. On average, though, people who fell ill had standard influenza symptoms—headache, fever, feeling weak, a sore throat, runny nose, and cough—that lasted for three or four days before they recovered. Even though the odds of experiencing the more severe effects were relatively low, the sheer number of people afflicted with the virus was statistically problematic for regions with limited medical resources. In October 1957, during the pandemic's peak in New York City, for example, there were more emergency calls than ambulances, and the city had to use unmarked cars to pick up the ill.

Science and Initiative to the Rescue

Previously, when the virus had raged in Hong Kong in April 1957, tens of thousands of people were hospitalized with complications from the Asian flu. Public awareness of the virus grew significantly as media outlets published pictures of Hong Kong's overflowing infirmaries.

To Maurice Hilleman, preparation for the impending pandemic included not just hospital beds but also an expedited vaccine. In large part due to Hilleman's initiatives, a vaccine was in production before the virus reached the United States in June 1957. Many scientists subsequently have praised Hilleman's foresight of the pandemic and contributions to virology throughout the twentieth century. In a 2011 interview, David M. Morens, a senior adviser to the director of the National Institute of Allergy and Infectious Diseases at the National Institutes of Health, said, "Unlike many scientists who understand the leaf on the tree, [Hilleman] understood the whole forest. And, of course, he also understood the leaf. He was one of the premier vaccinologists of the 20th century, and he really was a big picture guy."[2]

In addition to Hilleman's advocacy, the US government's effort to roll out the vaccine was also impressive. On September 2, 1957, *Life* magazine noted, "The government has launched the fastest medical mobilization ever attempted against an epidemic disease."[3] Many Americans were vaccinated in September, helping to slow the spread. Some foreign countries also developed vaccines to combat the disease. Others were less fortunate and simply endured the tragedy.

Early warning, Hilleman's initiative, and government funding of vaccine programs saved many lives from the ravages of the Asian flu. Because of scientific advancements in the study of viruses, pharmaceutical companies were able to work with government and civic leaders to contain a pandemic. Still, the disease held on for a decade in areas where resources were few. But by 1968, there were no more reported cases of the Asian flu in humans.

"The government has launched the fastest medical mobilization ever attempted against an epidemic disease."[3]

—*Life* magazine, September 2, 1957

CHAPTER ONE

A New Strain of Flu

In 1957, as Elvis Presley's "All Shook Up" played on the juke-box and Americans enjoyed *Old Yeller* at their local drive-in theaters, there was a notable atmosphere of unease. In the midst of the Cold War rivalry between the United States and the Soviet Union and their allies, many Americans grew concerned about another threat to public safety: a new strain of flu that was spreading worldwide like a fire across dry grass. Some even questioned whether the virus was naturally occurring or if, perhaps, it was a product of something more intentional and nefarious.

Alarmists believed weapons testing or biological warfare might have caused the new mystery flu or that the new virus was a consequence of nuclear testing in the Pacific. The fear was prevalent enough that US surgeon general Leroy E. Burney had to assure the nation that this was not the case. In response to the question of whether Communists had planted the virus, Burney said, "No. I don't believe that is a possibility. We have epidemics occasionally and have had them in the past."[4] Nonetheless, some Americans remained uncertain for months.

Origins and Media Attention

As it turns out, the surgeon general was correct. The virus did not come from nuclear testing or biological warfare. Rather, the Asian flu was the result of a mutation of a viral strain from wild ducks that combined with an existing human flu strain. The new virus was a subtype (H2N2) of influenza A, which is commonly associated with birds.

The mutated strain of influenza became known as the Asian flu because it arose somewhere in Asia, though there seem to be conflicting views on its exact origin. According to some historians, the first case was reported in the Guizhou province of southwestern China in 1956. From there, it spread as far as Singapore in February 1957. The Centers for Disease Control and Prevention (CDC), however, more vaguely claim the new virus originated in East Asia and was first reported in Singapore. In either case, the Asian flu eventually gained public notoriety in Singapore and became significant because of its symptoms, severe complications, death toll, and rapid spread.

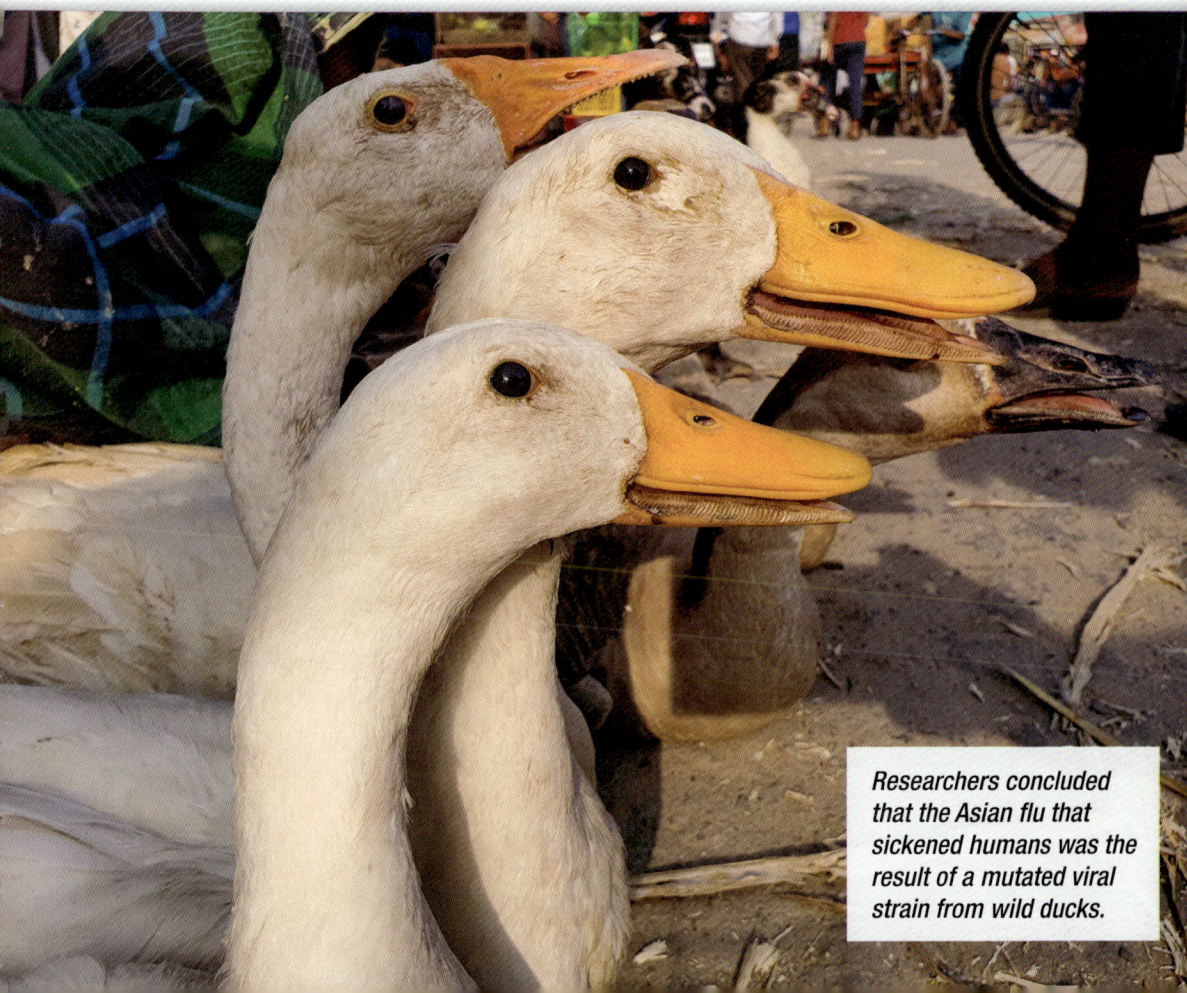

Researchers concluded that the Asian flu that sickened humans was the result of a mutated viral strain from wild ducks.

When the virus appeared in Singapore, it gained limited media attention. Singapore generally does not have well-defined flu seasons because of its tropical, rather than temperate, climate. Still, Singapore was not spared from the new virus. By May 7, 1957, the *Straits Times* declared that the Asian flu was "the worst in the Colony's [Singapore's] history."[5] The newspaper also reported that four times the usual number of children were absent from school the preceding day. In addition, during the Asian flu's peak in mid-May 1957 in Singapore, 47.6 percent of the 162,000 patients who went to medical clinics were being treated for influenza. The small country, with a population of only about 1.5 million at the time, experienced an accompanying increased mortality rate in May, accounting for an estimated 680 deaths from influenza.

Reporting on the new virus picked up considerably when it reached Hong Kong in April 1957. According to the *American Journal of Public Health*, the Asian flu entered Hong Kong via a refugee camp and might have been carried from people fleeing the interior of Communist China. Here again, the tracing of the spread is relatively uncertain given its unclear origins. But what is clear is that within the first days of its arrival in Hong Kong, the 700,000 people living in the close quarters of the refugee camp became sick. From there, the new virus spread rather quickly through Hong Kong, partly because of its dense population. At the time, Hong Kong had a population of 2.5 million people who lived on only 62 square miles (161 sq. km) of usable land. That month, the *New York Times* reported that 250,000 Hong Kong residents were being treated for influenza. The article described the impact on the young by noting that "many women carried glassy-eyed children tied to their backs."[6] Readers across the world were alarmed to learn about the inundation of Hong Kong's medical facilities with thousands of people standing in long lines for treatment of their symptoms.

"Many women [in Hong Kong] carried glassy-eyed children tied to their backs."[6]

—The *New York Times*, April 17, 1957

As the Asian flu spread across borders throughout Asia during the spring of 1957, it also affected an increasing number of people in the countries already contending with the virus. News stories grew more numerous and more worrisome. By May, for example, Reuters reported, "A Health Ministry Spokesman said the Singapore outbreak had reached epidemic proportions."[7]

The Symptoms of the New Virus

The new virus in Singapore and Hong Kong did not have symptoms that were substantially different from the seasonal flu. Rather, symptoms of the Asian flu were similar to those of other types of influenza. The people afflicted generally first experienced shaky legs and a chill. These symptoms were followed by an overall weakness, a sore throat, runny nose, cough, headache, and fever.

In June 1957, nine-year-old Sumi Krishna came down with the flu along with many of her classmates in Tamil Nadu, India. In May and June, 256 of the 533 students at Krishna's school (48 percent) had contracted the virus. Still, even while exhibiting symptoms, her school's headmaster allowed her to travel a day's journey by train to her grandparents' house. By the time she arrived, her fever had increased. She took to her bed, where she remained for a couple of weeks. The virus affected primarily her lungs, and with little appetite she lost weight. As a result of the virus, Krishna also had suffered eosinophilia, an increased number of white blood cells, which can lead to various disorders in affected organs. By July, despite the high infection rate, the school's newsletter had classified the virus as only a "mild epidemic."[8] This is likely because the symptoms in school-age children were comparable to seasonal influenza.

Adults and children tended to experience the virus a bit differently. Whereas adults were more likely to experience aching arms and legs, children often had headaches followed by a high fever (usually between 102°F and 104°F) lasting for about two days. Young children, particularly boys, experienced nosebleeds. Harvey Morris, who was eleven years old when he contracted the virus in the United States, explains, "A profuse nosebleed [is] what took me eventually by ambulance to the local emergency ward. Exciting! A kindly nurse stuffed my nostrils with bandage and after that I was on the mend."[9]

Severe Complications and Vulnerable Populations

Not all cases were as straightforward as Harvey Morris's. Three percent of those afflicted with the Asian flu experienced severe complications, about half of which were pneumonia and bronchitis. Other complications included seizures and heart failure. Some of these complications resulted in death. For example, following her recovery, Sumi Krishna learned that a twelve-year-old classmate from a nearby town in India had died from flu complications. As an adult, Krishna reflected on her classmate's death: "We were curious about who she was and why she had died while all of us had survived, but the teachers shushed the chatter."[10] By the time the new virus had swept across the subcontinent from May 1957 to February 1958, there were 4,451,758 cases, with 1,098 deaths reported in India.

The elderly, children under five years old, and pregnant women were particularly vulnerable to severe complications, including death, from the Asian flu. In total, there were an estimated 1.1 million to 2 million deaths (0.3 percent mortality rate) that resulted from the virus. The estimates vary because some people might have died because of complications from the virus but were never diagnosed. Alternatively, others who died after testing positive for the virus might have died even if they did not have it. The way in which people are counted in the death toll affects the numbers and mortality rate of the virus.

In contrast to the 0.3 percent mortality rate of the Asian flu, the estimated death rate of the seasonal flu today is 0.1 percent, according to Dr. Anthony Fauci, director of the US National Institute of Allergy and Infectious Diseases. The higher mortality rate in 1957 is likely due to how widespread the virus was, making

What's in a Name?

Sometimes names are controversial. The Asian flu was so named because it originated in East Asia. Other pandemics, such as the Russian flu or the Hong Kong flu, also have names tied to their origins. During the height of the Asian flu pandemic, there is little evidence to suggest that its naming sparked controversy. In the twenty-first century, however, there has been significant public backlash at naming viruses based on their origins. Looking back, Clark Whelton writes that the H2N2 virus was "known at the time by the politically incorrect name of 'Asian flu.'" Although not politically incorrect in 1957, it has become less acceptable over time to name a disease after a region because it tends to cast blame on those in that region for the disease and its consequences.

Naming practices change over time. In 2020 there was a public refusal to refer to COVID-19 as the "Chinese virus." Though it arose in China, there was concern that by associating the virus with an ethnicity, there would be an increased likelihood of blaming and victimizing Asians. Many people suggested that calling coronavirus the "Chinese virus" was not just a bad idea but a racist one.

Clark Whelton, "Say Your Prayers and Take Your Chances: Remembering the 1957 Asian Flu Pandemic," *City Journal*, March 13, 2020. www.city-journal.org.

vulnerable populations that much more susceptible to getting it. Additionally, advances in medicine and available hospital space in the absence of a pandemic tend to alleviate the death toll of the seasonal flu. The Asian flu pandemic overwhelmed medical services in many areas, drained medical supplies, and left many to perish from the lack.

A Variety of Victims

Among the casualties of the Asian flu in 1957 were people with fame, resources, and access to medical care. In November, two days after exhibiting symptoms of the new virus, opera singer Beniamino Gigli died from pneumonia at age sixty-seven in Milan, Italy. Gigli had been one of the most prominent and successful tenors of the 1920s through the 1940s. The *New York Times* reported, "At his bedside were his wife Costanza, his daughter, Rina with her husband, Lello Ceroni, his son, Renzo with his wife Wanda. A priest of Sinor Gigli's parish administered his last sacraments."[11]

About a month after Gigli died, famed American-born opera soprano Maria Callas also contracted the Asian flu in Italy. On January 2, 1958, Callas walked off the stage because she was sick during an unfinished gala performance in Rome. The audience and media were unforgiving of her early departure from the stage, and she was harshly criticized because the performance

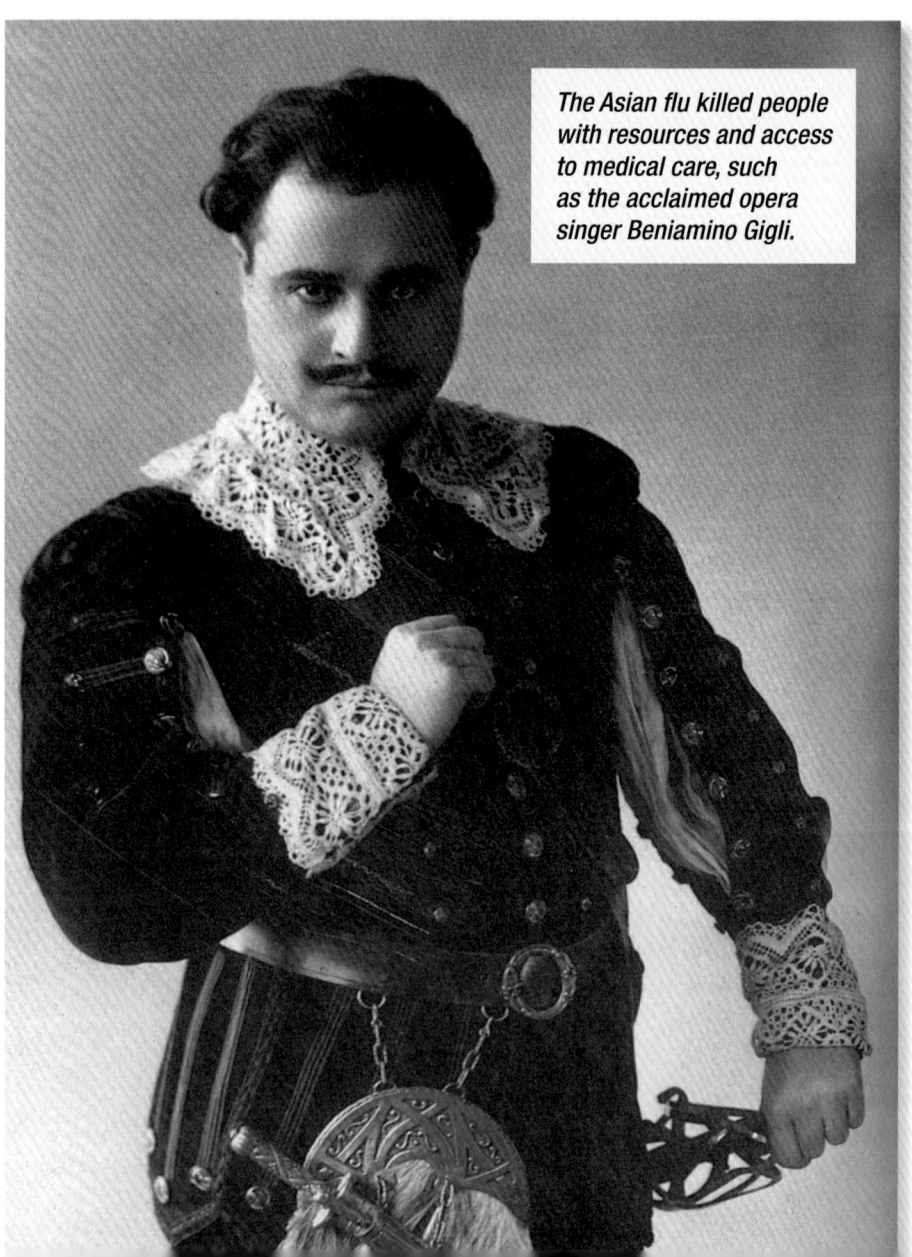

The Asian flu killed people with resources and access to medical care, such as the acclaimed opera singer Beniamino Gigli.

False Advertising

In the 1950s, there was a change in pharmaceutical marketing techniques that fostered false advertising. Drug firms once used their public relations offices to attract investors and maintain institutional publicity. After World War II, pharmaceutical companies began advertising directly to the public. By 1956 the leaders of pharmaceutical companies in the United States had organized to create the Health News Institute, a centralized public relations office for the pharmaceutical industry. With the rise of the Health News Institute, advertising techniques shifted from promoting firms to publicizing specific drugs directly to the people.

Given the heightened public concern associated with the Asian flu in 1957, drug firms were afforded a less-than-ethical, but lucrative, opportunity to market nasal sprays and mouthwashes that supposedly performed miracles. The institutional shift in marketing directly to the consumers at that time incentivized the pharmaceutical companies' false claims.

was suspended. Giovanni Gronchi, the president of Italy; his wife, Carla; and other members of Rome's high society were in attendance. Unlike Gigli, though, Callas did not suffer severe complications and made a complete recovery.

Although it was generally true that healthy people between ages five and sixty-five, such as Callas, did not suffer complications from the virus, there were some exceptions. For example, Paul Himmelman was a student at Colgate University when he contracted the Asian flu in October 1957. Himmelman, of Ossining, New York, who had competed on his high school track team, specializing in the 100- and 200-yard (91 and 183 m) races. By all reasonable predictions and health metrics, he should have recovered without complications from the virus. Sadly, he did not. On October 16, 1957, nineteen-year-old Himmelman died shortly after contracting the new influenza. Although the very young and old were usually the ones to suffer complications associated with the Asian flu, sometimes there were unknown factors or underlying medical conditions that explained how individuals, such as Himmelman, succumbed to the virus.

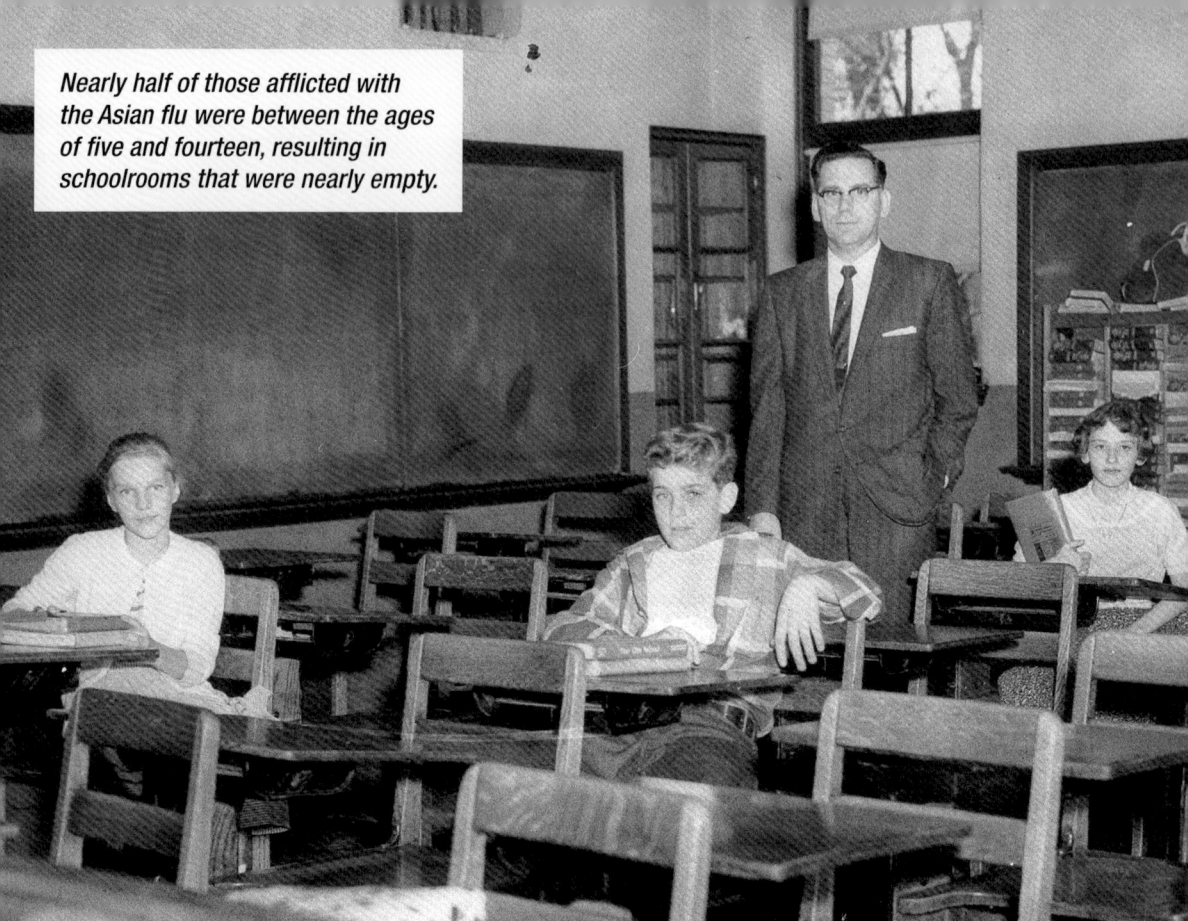

Fortunately, young children and the elderly—the most susceptible to severe complications—were not the majority of those who contracted the virus. Rather, most who got the Asian flu were between the ages of five and thirty-nine years old. In fact, 49 percent of those afflicted were between five and fourteen years old. This is likely due to the quick transmission of the new virus in schools. A 1959 report by the Government of India Influenza Centre at the Pasteur Institute supported this theory. It found that school-age children in India, particularly from ages six to ten, were the most likely population to contract the virus.

Treating the Symptoms

As a rising number of school-age children, their families, and others contracted the new virus across the world in 1957, they found that the easiest way to cope with the symptoms was to treat them as they would for other strains of the flu. They took to their beds to get plenty of rest, drank more fluids, and took over-the-counter medication to alleviate headaches and fever. In some cases, those afflicted had high fevers or trouble breathing, prompting them to seek medical care where available.

Clark Whelton, attending Bates College in Maine at the time, was among them. In October 1957, Whelton contracted the Asian flu. He later wrote, "My fever spiked to 105, and I was sicker than I'd ever been. The infirmary quickly filled with other cases, though some ailing students toughed it out in their dorm rooms with aspirin and orange juice."[12] Whelton recovered completely from his illness.

Shortly after Whelton's illness, on November 1, 1957, the *New York Times* reported that the flu and pneumonia toll in the United States was 2.5 times higher than it had been during the previous year. There was some concern among the American public. The masses were not yet vaccinated, and people had been reading about the impending new influenza virus for about seven months in the newspapers.

Opportunistic pharmaceutical companies saw a marketing opportunity to leverage fear for financial gains. Some of them were making unrealistic promises about their products' capabilities. A November 1957 US Food and Drug Administration (FDA) report stated, "We are distressed . . . by the sheer opportunism of some drug firms which are knowingly and purposely misleading the public by attempting to make them believe that the use of this or that proprietary preparation will provide them with a significant

> "My fever spiked to 105, and I was sicker than I'd ever been. The infirmary quickly filled with other cases, though some ailing students toughed it out in their dorm rooms with aspirin and orange juice."[12]
>
> —Clark Whelton, who contracted Asian flu as a college student in October 1957

> "We are distressed . . . by the sheer opportunism of some drug firms which are knowingly and purposely misleading the public."[13]
>
> —US Food and Drug Administration report, November 1957

degree of protection against the Asian flu."[13] As a result, the FDA issued a warning that it would take action against companies that claimed their products (such as mouthwashes or nose and throat sprays) would prevent or cure the Asian flu.

In the end, the only method to prevent acquiring the new virus was vaccination. Before that eventuality, the disease continued to spread easily and rapidly across porous borders. Citizens of all nations followed the news of its journey and the stories of sickness and overcrowded medical facilities left in its wake. Its magnitude, both in terms of the virus's rapid transmission and mortality rate, had not been witnessed for about forty years. For most people who contracted the Asian flu, its destruction as an influenza virus was unprecedented in their lifetimes.

CHAPTER TWO

The Rise of the Pandemic

On May 12, 1957, the SS *Rajula*, a large steamship carrying 1,622 travelers and 200 crew members, docked at the port of Madras on the southeastern coast of India. Many aboard the ship, which had sailed from Singapore, were already suffering from the Asian flu. The *Rajula* may not have been the only means by which the H2N2 virus entered the subcontinent, but it has become the most noted. Regardless, by June 1957, there were over 1 million cases of Asian flu throughout India. During the summer of 1957, Sushila Nayar, a politician, medical doctor, and former health minister of India, observed, "Conditions are very bad. There are whole families lying sick and there is nobody to give them even water. Nobody has taken steps to see that there are emergency beds, emergency measures are taken and something is done to take care of the people. This is so in many parts of India."[14]

The overall population and its density in India provided many viral hosts and quick avenues for the new disease to spread throughout the nation. India's example convinced some international organizations and governments to realize that the world was not simply dealing with a traditional seasonal flu but something more substantial.

An Epidemic Becomes a Pandemic

On June 7, 1957, the World Health Organization (WHO)—the United Nations agency mandated to coordinate international responses to health crises—still referred to the Asian flu as a mild epidemic of influenza because the new strain of H2N2 seemed to be restricted to a relatively small region of the globe. However, it did not take long until WHO and others recognized it as a pandemic that spreads over continents. Even by June, the Asian flu had spread from East Asia to Australia and Indonesia in addition to India. By the end of the month, the pandemic was in western Europe, North America, Pakistan, and the Middle East. The virus further traveled to South America, South Africa, New Zealand, and the Pacific Islands in July. It continued to eastern Europe, the rest of Africa, and the Caribbean in August. The Asian flu pandemic had covered the world in about six months.

Some pandemics are more serious in symptoms, mortality rates, and contagion than others depending on virus mutation and antibodies in the population. Influenza pandemics occur about every ten to eleven years with a viral mutation of the annual seasonal influenza. The biology of contagion is the same for seasonal influenza and influenza pandemics. Influenza is spread either by contact or by droplets of mucus or saliva cast out into the air when an afflicted person coughs or sneezes. When there is a genetic mutation in the flu strain, however, a higher percentage of the population is susceptible to the mutated flu because it does not have the antibodies for immunity. The only people known

"Conditions are very bad. There are whole families lying sick and there is nobody to give them even water. Nobody has taken steps to see that there are emergency beds, emergency measures are taken and something is done to take care of the people."[14]

—Sushila Nayar, a member of the Indian Parliament from 1957 to 1971

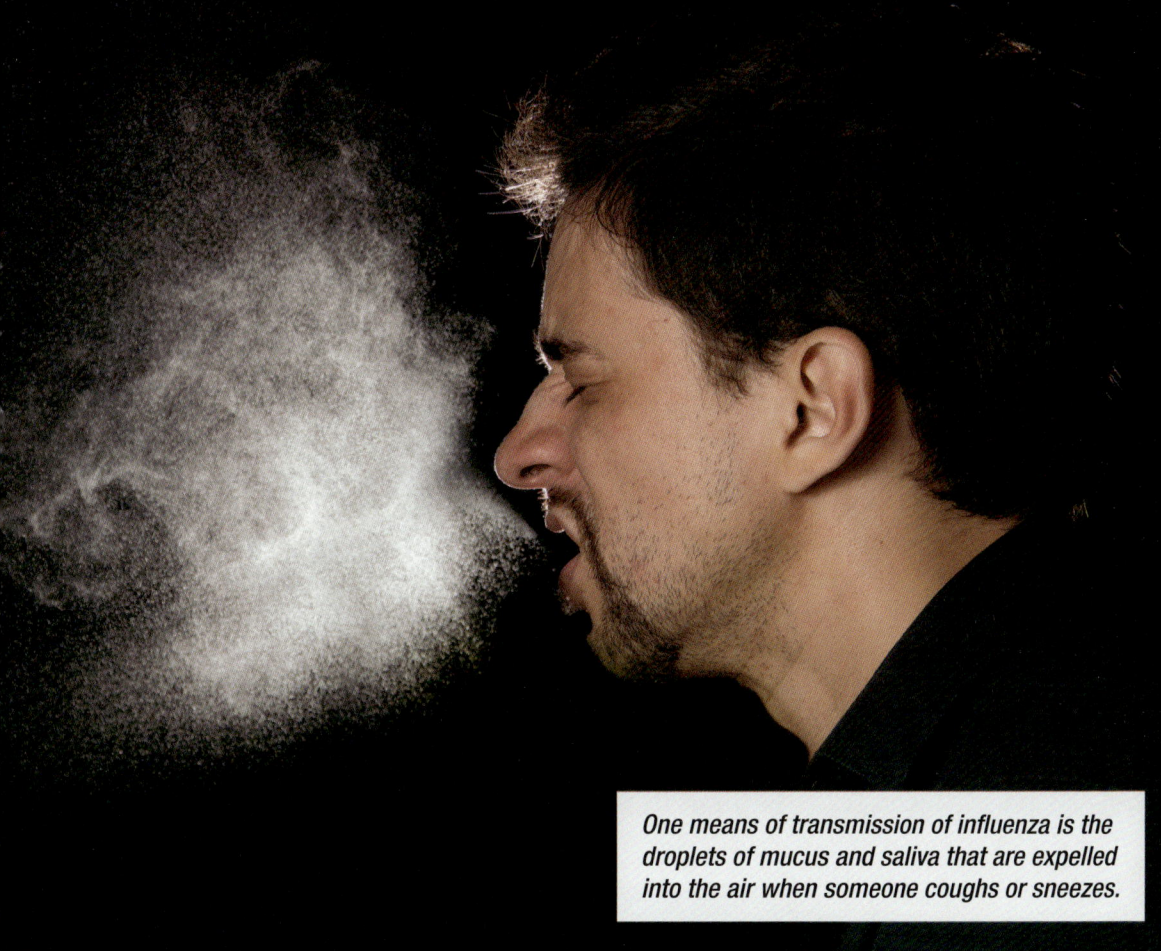

One means of transmission of influenza is the droplets of mucus and saliva that are expelled into the air when someone coughs or sneezes.

to be immune to the Asian flu of 1957 were those who, about seven decades prior, had contracted and survived the Russian flu virus of 1889. Thus, there were not many people immune to the pandemic of 1957.

Spread over Land and Sea

The potential hosts for the Asian flu, scattered across the world, generally came into contact with the pandemic as a result of their contact with other people during land and sea, rather than air, travel. Jet passenger travel first began in 1952. Five years on, in 1957, airplanes were a much less typical means of travel in comparison to ships, trains, and cars. The seats were bigger then, with more leg room, and flight attendants served full meals on real

Virus Spreads to World Leaders but Spares President Eisenhower

World leaders were also contracting the pandemic while public health officials and politicians alike were working together to understand and contain it. Sixty-four-year-old Syrian president Shukri al-Kuwatli contracted the virus at a diplomatic reception in July 1957. On July 15, Reuters reported that five thousand cases of Asian flu had been reported in Damascus, Syria.

On October 7, 1957, the *New York Times* reported that across the world the pandemic was spreading rapidly in Brazil. Brazil would contend with the Asian flu for years to come. In February 1960, Brazilian president Juscelino Kubitschek fell ill with the virus and had a high fever. On his doctor's advice, Kubitschek canceled all of his appointments in the following weeks, which included a meeting with US president Dwight Eisenhower.

President Eisenhower's chief economic adviser, Gabriel Hauge, also fell ill with the Asian flu and exhibited symptoms only shortly after a meeting with the president in late August 1957. President Eisenhower had been vaccinated against the virus only six days prior but did not contract the flu during his meeting with Hauge.

china plates, but the prices were cost-prohibitive for most people. During the mid-1950s, a bargain fare seat on a one-way flight from New York to Paris was roughly $2,600 in modern currency. During the 1950s, there were fewer than 100,000 air travelers arriving to or departing from the United States on an average day. In contrast, there were approximately 2.5 million air travelers per day going through airport checkpoints in 2019. Most international travelers in 1957 were still getting from place to place by train or car or aboard ships such as the SS *Rajula*.

The Spread of Asian Flu in the United States

Some of the first reported cases in the United States were among the crews of several destroyers (warships) at Newport Naval Station in Rhode Island in June 1957. There were also early cases among navy recruits in San Diego and army recruits at Fort Ord, California. Some of them had contracted the Asian flu in Hong Kong. It was particularly consequential that members of the navy had the Asian flu because viruses tend to spread quickly among people aboard ships and on naval bases with tight living quarters. Navy service-members also carried the virus to the ports at which they were docked. On June 22, 1957, the *New York Times* reported that 550 sailors among eight naval ships had contracted the virus.

Some civilians also were exposed to the virus while traveling internationally to the United States. In early June, there were also 96 cases of the Asian flu reported on the passenger steamship the *President Cleveland*, which was crossing from the Philippines to San Francisco. Nine-year-old Joye Jones was on the ship traveling with her parents, who had been missionaries in Burma. She later recalled, "I do remember many people getting sick on board, although it wasn't until we were approaching Oakland that I found

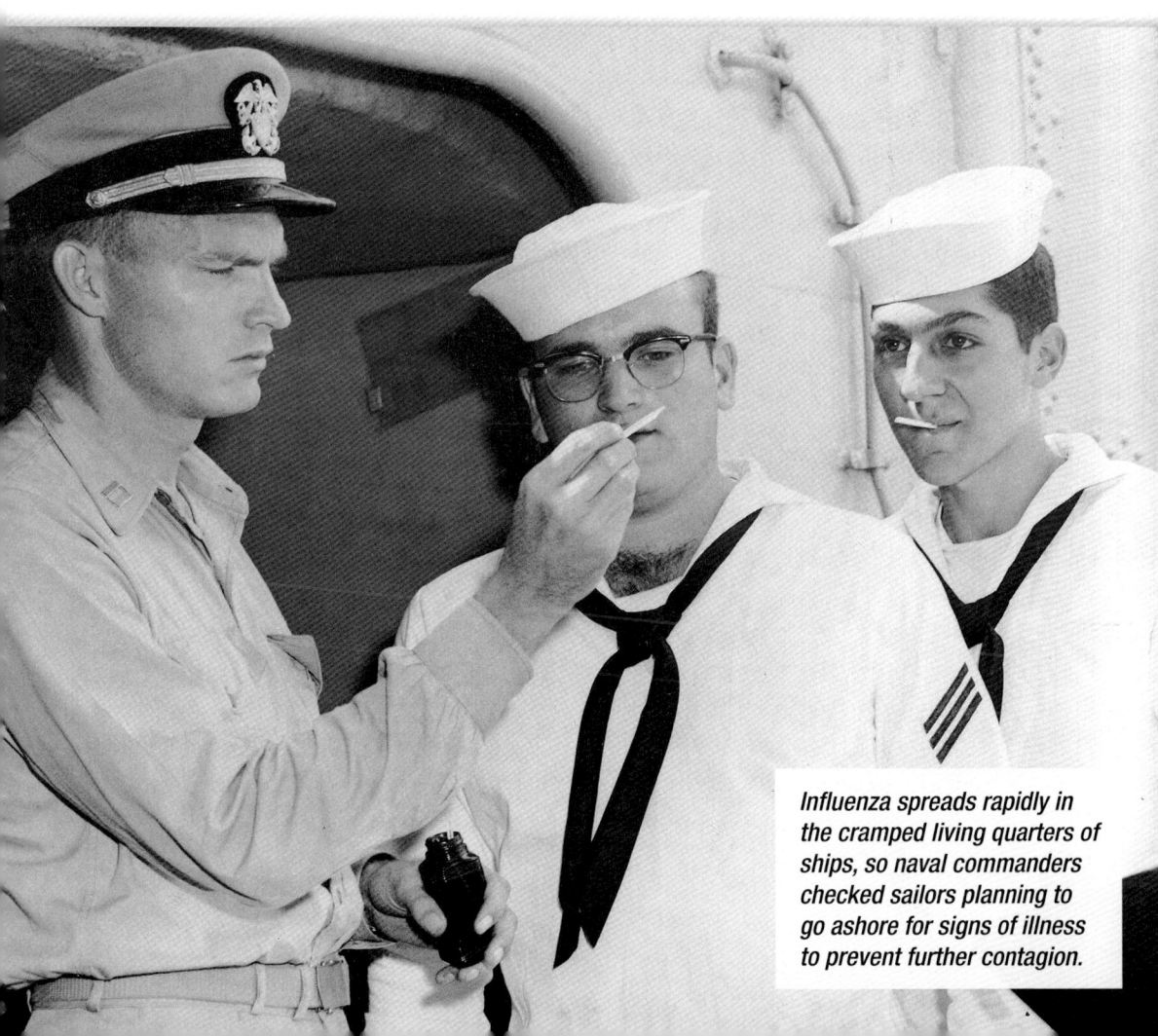

Influenza spreads rapidly in the cramped living quarters of ships, so naval commanders checked sailors planning to go ashore for signs of illness to prevent further contagion.

out it was the flu. My parents worried that we would be quarantined on board because so many people were ill. But for whatever reason, we docked and disembarked on schedule. We then took the train across the U.S. to Mississippi where my grandparents lived. By the time we arrived, so had the flu."[15] From the coastal cities, the virus moved inland with international as well as domestic travelers.

Gatherings Provide Many Viral Hosts

At the end of June 1957, for example, a high school student from California traveled to Grinnell, Iowa, to attend a Presbyterian youth meeting at Grinnell College. She developed symptoms on her way there and exposed 1,680 delegates from over forty states and ten other countries to the virus. The *New York Times* reported on July 2, 1957, that 200 of the delegates contracted the flu. The meeting was canceled with two days remaining. Those presenting symptoms were treated at Grinnell College's medical facility, and the rest of the attendees were sent home early on buses and trains. Dr. Tom Chin, a representative from the US Public Health Service's Communicable Disease Center at Kansas City, had traveled to Grinnell to survey the situation. In defense of sending the conference attendees home, he said, "Permitting the young people to travel to their homes will not prove to be a great problem. . . . The illness is not serious. It runs about two days."[16] Attendees of the youth meeting subsequently spread the virus to many previously unaffected areas of the United States.

> "Permitting the young people to travel to their homes will not prove to be a great problem. . . . The illness is not serious. It runs about two days."[16]
>
> —Dr. Tom Chin, a representative from the US Public Health Service's Communicable Disease Center in Kansas City

Similarly, throughout July and August 1957, there were reports of Boy Scout groups traveling around the country and inadvertently spreading the virus as well. In early July, Camp Roosevelt, a Boy Scout camp near Chesapeake Beach, Maryland, closed

Mortality and the Asian Flu in Chile

Santiago, Chile, with a 1.99 percent mortality rate, was one of the cities hit hardest by the virus. Throughout Chile, people were dying in comparatively large numbers. On August 19, 1957, *Time* magazine reported, "Funeral homes sold out their coffins, and queues waited in cemeteries with their dead while laborers dug graves." On one day alone in the summer of 1957, there were two hundred deaths from flu complications—a significant amount in a country with a population of 6.9 million people.

As the Asian flu pandemic of 1957 spread across the world, it became clear that mortality rates varied across nations. A study in the *Journal of Infectious Diseases* found that, on average, countries in Latin America experienced the highest rates of death from the pandemic, whereas nations in Europe experienced the lowest. Academic speculation on mortality rate ranges for the Asian flu pandemic generally focuses on the wealth of nations, citizens' access to medical care, and the age distribution of the population.

Time, "Chile: The Flu Spreads," August 19, 1957, vol. 70, no. 8.

when seventy campers came down with the flu. Around the same time, from July 11 to 18, Valley Forge, Pennsylvania, hosted the International Boy Scout Jamboree. There were fifty-three thousand participants, including the Scouts and leaders, from every state and several countries. From the beginning of the event, attendees from California, Louisiana, and Puerto Rico had exhibited symptoms of what turned out to be the Asian flu. Events like the International Boy Scout Jamboree and the Presbyterian meeting at Grinnell College quickened the virus's spread inland.

With an exponential growth in viral spread throughout the nation, in August 1957 Surgeon General Burney warned that the autumn would bring a "sweeping and widespread" outbreak throughout the nation. He asserted, "There will not be enough time, of course, to produce and administer sufficient vaccine to immunize a majority of the population before the influenza season."[17]

The surgeon general was right. As predicted, the number of Asian flu cases in the United States continued to increase with the opening of schools and colleges in early September 1957. On October 2, the New York City Health Department reported that 150,000 pupils (20 percent of enrollment) and three thousand teachers had contracted the Asian flu. Absenteeism in some schools across the nation reached levels of 30 to 50 percent. Throughout the autumn of 1957, numbers were on the rise across the entire country.

Cases in Europe

Global transmission patterns paralleled those in the United States during the summer and autumn of 1957. On June 4, 1957, around the same time that the Asian flu arrived in the United States via ships, it made landfall in western Europe. A person carrying the virus traveled on an airplane from Jakarta, Indonesia, to the Netherlands. On June 16, an unrelated case was detected in the Netherlands at a girls' school near Amsterdam. The second case was thought to have originated from ships arriving at ports in Rotterdam and the Hague. Like the Americans' experience with the pandemic, throughout the summer, large outbreaks of the virus occurred in crowded communities in the Netherlands and as it traveled through Europe.

Whereas land route transmission in the United States primarily spread from two large events—the Presbyterian meeting in Grinnell and the Boy Scout jamboree in Pennsylvania—the Asian flu made its way through much of Europe on land routes from Russia to Scandinavia and eastern Europe. It had entered the Union of Soviet Socialist Republics (USSR) in the beginning of May 1957 via neighboring countries. Initially, during the early summer months, cases were documented only in certain cities, such as Tashkent (Uzbekistan), Stalinabad (now Dushanbe, Turkmenistan), Ashkabad (Turkmenistan), and other places in Central Asia. During the later summer and fall months—when the Soviets released *Sputnik 1*, the first artificial satellite, into space—the Asian flu spread throughout all regions of the USSR. The pandemic traveled throughout the USSR and into neighboring countries and eventually Scandinavia along the Trans-Siberian Railway, the longest railway line in the world.

In August 1957, Scandinavian attendees of a youth festival in Moscow, who had traveled part of their way on the Trans-Siberian Railway, brought the virus home with them. The pandemic went through Sweden within weeks as it spread through schools, workplaces, and camps. High rates of absences were reported in the postal and telegraphic services, the national railway company, and schools. By the end of 1958, an estimated 15 percent of the Swedish population had contracted the virus, but the mortality rate was lower than the global average, 0.2 percent.

In the summer of 1957, the new virus was in full effect in the United Kingdom as well. The pandemic had entered England in June, where among the first cases was a young Hungarian refugee admitted to a hospital in Birmingham with symptoms of the Asian flu. There was a full outbreak across the United Kingdom in August, with spiraling contagion associated with schoolchildren, and a peak in the middle of October.

In the United Kingdom, doctors held conflicting opinions of the pandemic's severity. After running its course, it had infected 9 to 12 million and killed 33,000 Britons, with three times the mortality rate of the seasonal flu of the previous year. Still, while some doctors believed it constituted a public health crisis, others did not. On the one hand, a British general practitioner later reflecting on the pandemic stated, "We were amazed at the extraordinary infectivity of the disease, overawed by the suddenness of its outset and surprised at the protean [changeable] nature of its symptomatology."[18] On the other hand, Dr. Douglas Cusiter, Yorkshire's medical officer of health, criticized media for spreading alarm over the virus. Cusiter argued that public health labs were forced to spend their resources examining influenza germs when they should have been focusing on poliomyelitis,

> "We were amazed at the extraordinary infectivity of the disease, overawed by the suddenness of its outset and surprised at the protean nature of its symptomatology."[18]
>
> —A British general practitioner

a crippling contagious disease that was also rampant during the 1950s. He claimed that the Asian flu was "a mild illness and a short one. The only thing new about it is that we have not had this strain of this influenza in this country before."[19]

Asian Flu in the Middle East and Africa

The novelty of virus and its contagiousness had worldwide consensus, even if concern for its severity did not. By July 1957, the pandemic had reached Saudi Arabia, Kuwait, Yemen, Syria, Iran, Iraq, and Jordan. Many pilgrims to the holy city of Mecca in Saudi Arabia contracted the virus and brought it back to their home countries and spread it to others en route. For example, on July 15, 1957, a Jordanian government spokesman reported that the pandemic arrived in Jordan by Pakistani Muslim pilgrims passing through on their way to Mecca.

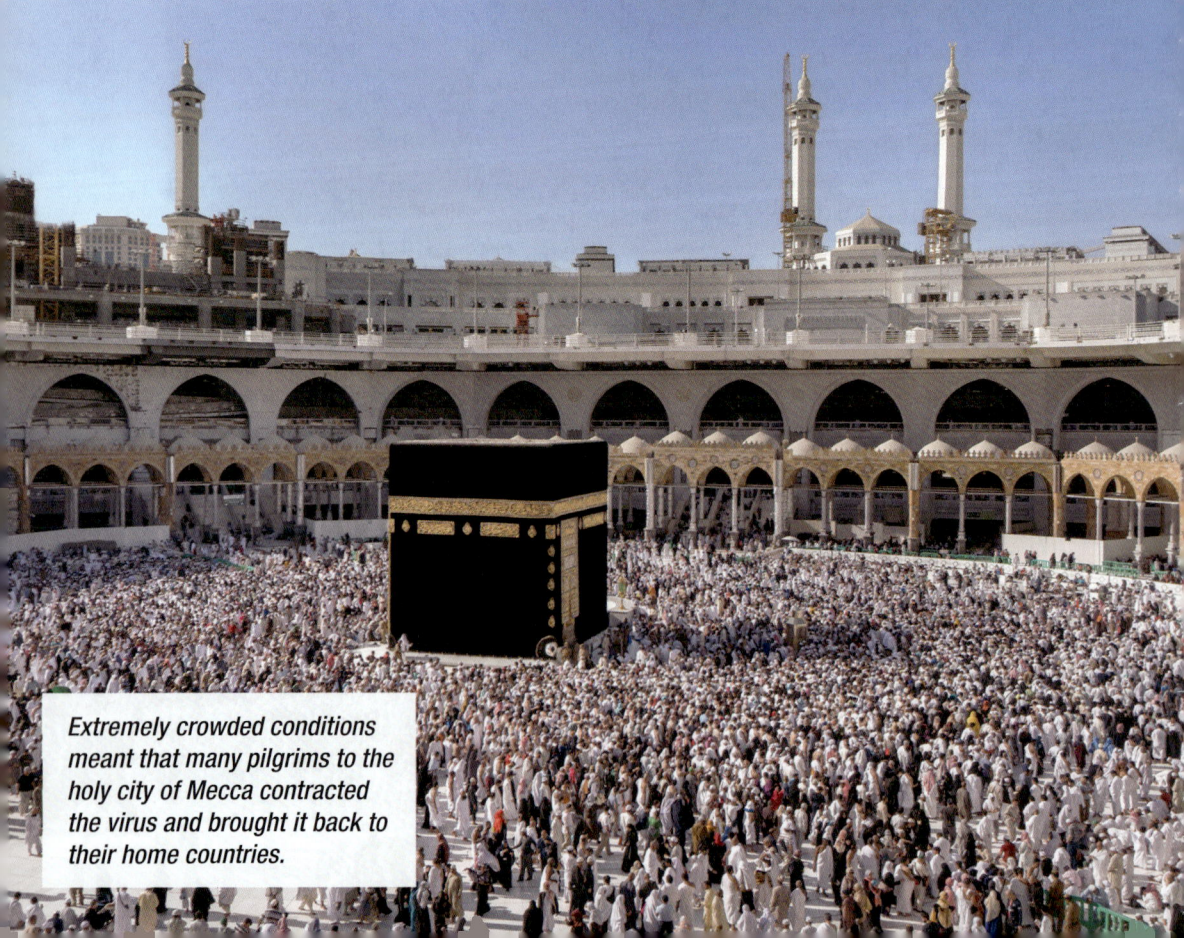

Extremely crowded conditions meant that many pilgrims to the holy city of Mecca contracted the virus and brought it back to their home countries.

In early August 1957, the Asian flu reached Kano, Nigeria, also by way of Muslim pilgrims returning by airplane from Mecca. By September 1, the city of Lagos reportedly had been crippled with shutdowns from the quick spread of the illness. The pandemic further continued to spread via land routes through West Africa as it made its way into Ghana and neighboring countries.

By the time Lagos suffered an outbreak, East African countries had already been infected with the pandemic primarily via land routes from the Middle East. On July 28, 1957, the USS *Rooks*, an American naval destroyer, arrived in Italy from its military supply base port in Massawa, Eritrea, in East Africa. The ship had to be quarantined. There were twenty-one servicemen aboard the ship with fever cases thought to be Asian flu. As the world's nations became increasingly saturated with pandemic victims, tracing the origins of the virus became more difficult. Initially, governments and health organizations could follow the course of the contagion from specific dockings or other travel routes in hopes of limiting the spread, but now the large number of international travelers were adding cases to nations that already had many.

Influenza rarely becomes a pandemic comparable to the scope and magnitude of the Asian flu. There was an almost eerie quiet before the viral storm of 1957. John Corbett McDonald, a pioneering British researcher in the field of epidemiology, noted in his quarterly report to the Royal College of General Practitioners that during the winter months of 1956 and early 1957, there was a "remarkably low level of respiratory illness so far this winter."[20] Given the pandemic that took over the world shortly afterward, it seems this was the quiet before the storm.

CHAPTER THREE

Containing the Spread

On October 13, 1957, hundreds of flyers rained down from an airplane flying over Mount Holyoke College, a women's college in South Hadley, Massachusetts. Students at Mount Holyoke were under quarantine as a new influenza pandemic was spreading around the world. Classes were canceled, and the gymnasium was being used to treat the people who had fallen ill. Lillian Hann Young was on one of the gymnasium cots that morning when she heard the buzz of the airplane and the commotion of her fellow students. According to the *Mount Holyoke News*, "Crowds of eager women defy high heels and tight skirts, dash to the field, clutch fiercely for the bits of comfort, smile serenely, contentedly as to their wondering eyes appear: YALE-MT. HOLYOKE AIRLIFT."[21] Printed on the flyers was a message from male students at nearby Yale University: "We hope the scourge of this virus will soon be erased from your fair campus and the quarantine lifted. . . . Keep smiling. We are thinking of you and we shall return."[22]

During the Asian flu pandemic, colleges like Mount Holyoke, public schools, hospitals, and governments across the world had to make decisions about whether or not they would be proactive in preventing the spread of the virus. The Asian flu was widely recognized to be highly contagious but not particularly deadly. Moreover, there were measures here and there to prevent spread in certain localities, but not much in terms of systematic policy across nations. For example, a few local governments in the United States restricted public gatherings. Meanwhile, some hospitals regulated visitor policies for patients. One of the main methods local government officials used to prevent the spread of the Asian flu in the United States and other nations was to close schools.

Deciding Whether to Close Schools in the United States

It became clear that the pandemic was spreading significantly as children returned to their schools in the fall of 1957. Children congregated in classrooms, cafeterias, and gymnasiums, where they shared their germs and then brought them home to their parents and families. As Asian flu cases increased, some districts decided to take action to try to prevent the spread. For example, school districts such as Fairfax County, the largest school district in Virginia, closed public schools.

In contrast, New York City's schools remained open. On October 8, 1957, the *New York Times* reported that 29 percent of the city's 280,164 students were not in their classes. The mayor's

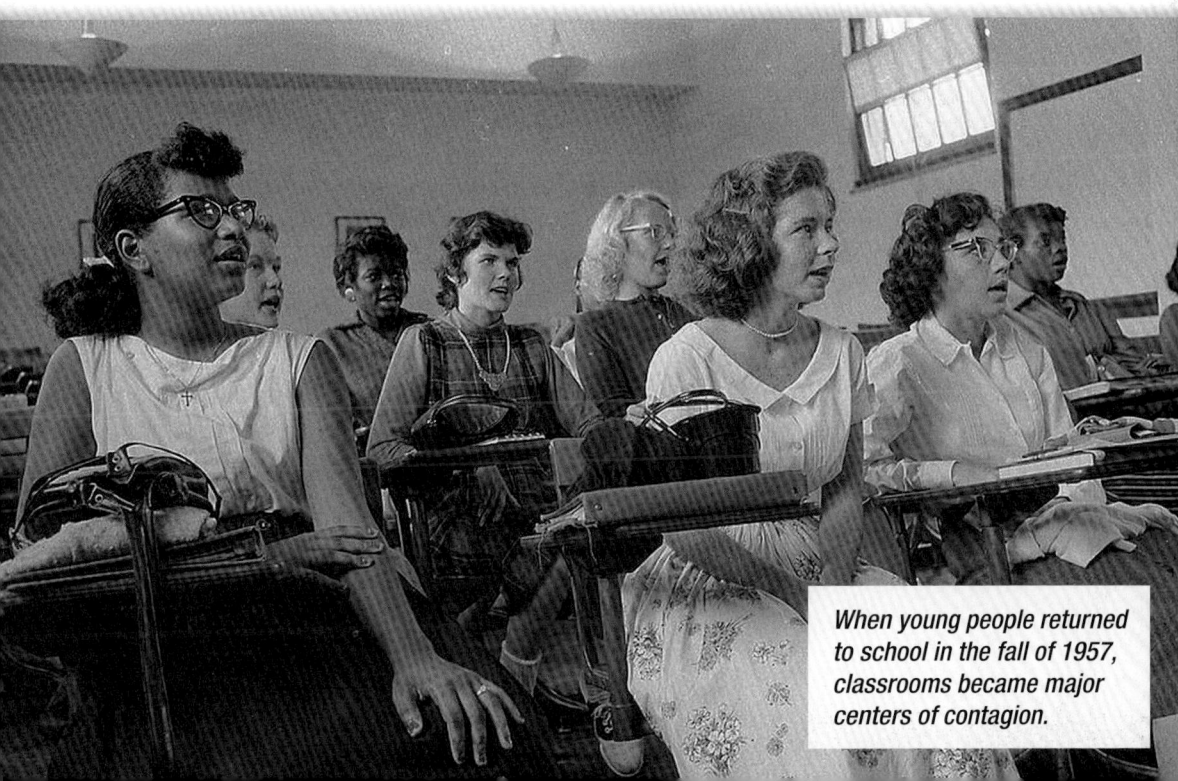

When young people returned to school in the fall of 1957, classrooms became major centers of contagion.

office further reported that over a five-day period in early October 1957, about eleven thousand people visited fifteen area hospitals with flu-like symptoms. Despite hospital visits and widespread cases in schools at that time, Dr. Roscoe Kandle, the acting New York City health commissioner, emphasized the relative mildness of the virus. He claimed, "[The Asian flu] is mild, the fever lasting about 48 hours. Many who have been stricken have already recovered."[23]

When the virus moved to upstate New York in October 1957, public officials took a different approach from their urban counterparts. They closed sixty schools, leaving about thirty-two thousand students out of their classrooms. Not all of them agreed that this was the best measure. Following a football game cancellation, the *Schenectady Gazette* reported that Dr. Malcolm A. Bouton, the health commissioner of Scotia, New York, said that "he would not advise closing schools or stopping any additional athletic contests or other public assemblies as a preventative measure. The commissioner adds there is no indication that closing schools or halting meetings would have any effect on the spread of the flu."[24]

Earlier in the year, public officials had reached a similar conclusion. On August 27 and 28, Surgeon General Burney had held meetings for state and local health officers in Washington, DC, and Bethesda, Maryland, to discuss the pandemic. At these meetings, the Community Planning Committee stated, "There is no practical advantage in the closing of schools or the curtailment of public gatherings. However, in some instances there may be administrative reasons for closing schools due to illness of teachers, bus drivers, large absentee rates, and so forth."[25]

"There is no practical advantage in the closing of schools or the curtailment of public gatherings. However, in some instances there may be administrative reasons for closing schools due to illness of teachers, bus drivers, large absentee rates, and so forth."[25]

—The US surgeon general's Community Planning Committee during an August 1957 meeting

Closing Schools in Other Countries

Some public officials worldwide, however, believed that closing the schools would contain the pandemic's spread. In northern Japan, for example, there was an Asian flu outbreak in the spring of 1960. Nearly fifty-one thousand cases were reported, leading to twenty-three deaths. As a result, officials there closed hundreds of schools. This was not the first time the country had experienced school closures for the Asian flu pandemic. In Tokyo in June 1957, an estimated seventy thousand children were afflicted with the flu, and eighty-seven schools were closed in response.

Similarly, in some areas of the United Kingdom, schools were closed during the pandemic. Research suggests that in the case of the Asian flu pandemic, children, who accounted for only 13 percent of the population in the United Kingdom, were responsible for 30 to 40 percent of the nation's infections. One day during the pandemic's peak, 110,000 of London's schoolchildren were absent from classes.

There is no consensus regarding the effects of school closures during a pandemic. Although children are not with their classmates when school is closed, their exposure to other children might not be reduced significantly if they are in child care centers, play sports, or hang out with other neighborhood children while they are not in school. At what point in the pandemic a school shuts down is also important in determining the extent to which closures will affect the spread. An earlier shutdown would likely be more productive than a later one when numbers are already high.

Restrictions on Public Gatherings and Hospital Visitation

Just as some officials were hesitant to close schools, there were few governmental restrictions on public gatherings. When there were limitations, they were implemented at the local, rather than state or national, level. Furthermore, restrictions on gatherings

The Media's Mixed Messages

Media reporting and representation of a pandemic influences the public's response. There was no doubt that the Asian flu was traveling around the world quickly and making people sick. But there were questions about how dangerous the virus was, how much people should worry, and what precautions they should take. In 1957 people were getting mixed messages from their newspapers. While discouraging panic, most newspapers ran continuous headlines about an increase of flu cases and death. Yet within those same papers might be articles that downplayed the crisis. On June 6, for example, the *Birmingham Daily Post* reported that ministers "stress there is no cause for alarm as the 'flu' germ is of a perfectly ordinary variety resulting in temperatures which last two or three days." Readers across the world were receiving both types of messages almost daily. The varied reporting on the pandemic created fear and uncertainty and inspired one newspaper humorist to write, "Fever is the second part of Asian flu. The first part is worse. That's the shivers you get from all the advance warnings."

Quoted in Freddie Attenborough, "The 1957–58 Asian Flu Pandemic: Why Did the UK Respond So Differently?," Lockdown Sceptics, June 5, 2020. https://lockdownsceptics.org.

Quoted in John Kelly, "In 1957, a New Flu Appeared in Asia. The World Watched and Waited for It to Spread," *Washington Post*, March 17, 2020. www.washingtonpost.com.

seemed to be the exception rather than the rule. High school football games were canceled here and there in October in upstate New York. In Maine, though, Clark Whelton reports playing an intercollegiate soccer game on the day he was released from the infirmary after recovering from the Asian flu. Collegiate sports also continued normally during the pandemic with full spectatorship. The college football season culminated with the Iowa Hawkeyes beating the Oregon State Beavers in the 1957 Rose Bowl in Pasadena, California, in front of approximately ninety-seven thousand live spectators.

In Cochise County, Arizona, however, restrictions were more severe. In August 1957, the pandemic had first appeared in one of the state's prisons in Pinal County, where 75–100 prisoners presented flu-like symptoms. By mid-September there was another outbreak of 225 cases of (suspected, not confirmed) Asian flu in neighboring Cochise County at Fort Huachuca. In response, the county closed all places of public gathering. The policy did little to slow the spread throughout the state, though. On September 25, 1957, Arizona's health commissioner reported that the transmission of the virus had reached epidemic levels. It is unclear, however, whether citizens respected the restrictions or found other ways to gather on their own.

With increasing infection levels, some hospitals across the United States changed visitor regulations during the pandemic to prevent an overwhelming demand for medical treatment. District of Columbia General Hospital, for example, restricted visitors to patients' immediate families and encouraged all well-wishers to send letters instead of visiting. In Schenectady, New York, three hospitals were completely closed to visitors in mid-October 1957 when twenty thousand people in the area were being treated for flu symptoms. Though it seems intuitive that keeping visitors away from flu patients would prevent some spread, the act was not enough to make a dent in the region's cases. Flu numbers surged in Schenectady County by the end of October, and only three of seven school districts remained open.

Ineffective Screening Measures for Travelers

Countries and regions varied in their willingness to close schools and limit public gatherings, but all seemed less inclined to restrict travel. There were very few travel restrictions barring afflicted people from traveling during the pandemic. In June 1957 Surgeon General Burney worked with the Advisory Committee on Influenza to draft a preparedness plan to mitigate the effects of the pandemic. As one of the preventive measures, Burney ordered quarantine officers to be posted at West Coast seaports and airports to monitor the situation. The Quarantine Service found that the Asian flu did not require quarantine. The US Public Health Service, which houses the Quarantine Service, stated, "The disease thus far has been mild, with most cases having only three or four days of fever. The death toll in the Far East is not considered high in view of the large numbers stricken."[26]

Moreover, these officers did not quarantine travelers who presented symptoms of the Asian flu on the West Coast. Rather, they checked some incoming ships and planes to see if there were suspected cases of the pandemic. The quarantine officers then sent the contact information of people who had respiratory illnesses to the health officers of the communities to which those individuals were traveling. This preparedness plan did nothing to prevent the spread of the virus but did allow quarantine officers the ability to trace its journey through the United States.

Similarly, public officials in Turkey were concerned about the pandemic's spread but did little to contain it. By July 1957, the pandemic had reached Iran, Iraq, and Syria at the borders of Turkey. Public officials had their eyes on the potential spread from pilgrims to and from Mecca, by large volumes of land traffic over the shared border with Iran and via trade routes over the Turkish-Syrian border. To address the impending threat, in late July 1957 the Turkish Ministry of Health and Social Welfare sent public health specialists to cities on the southeastern border. They took throat swabs and sent them to Ankara, the nation's capital, for laboratory investigation. By late August 1957, cases of the Asian flu were reported in almost all regions of Turkey.

That same month, officials in the Netherlands prohibited forty-four Turkish exchange students from boarding the ship *Arosa Sky*, which was sailing from Rotterdam to the United States. Fifteen of the students had the flu. They ended up flying to New York City instead, and three of them required medical treatment when they arrived. The

"The disease thus far has been mild, with most cases having only three or four days of fever. The death toll in the Far East is not considered high in view of the large numbers stricken."[26]

—The US Public Health Service in 1957

38

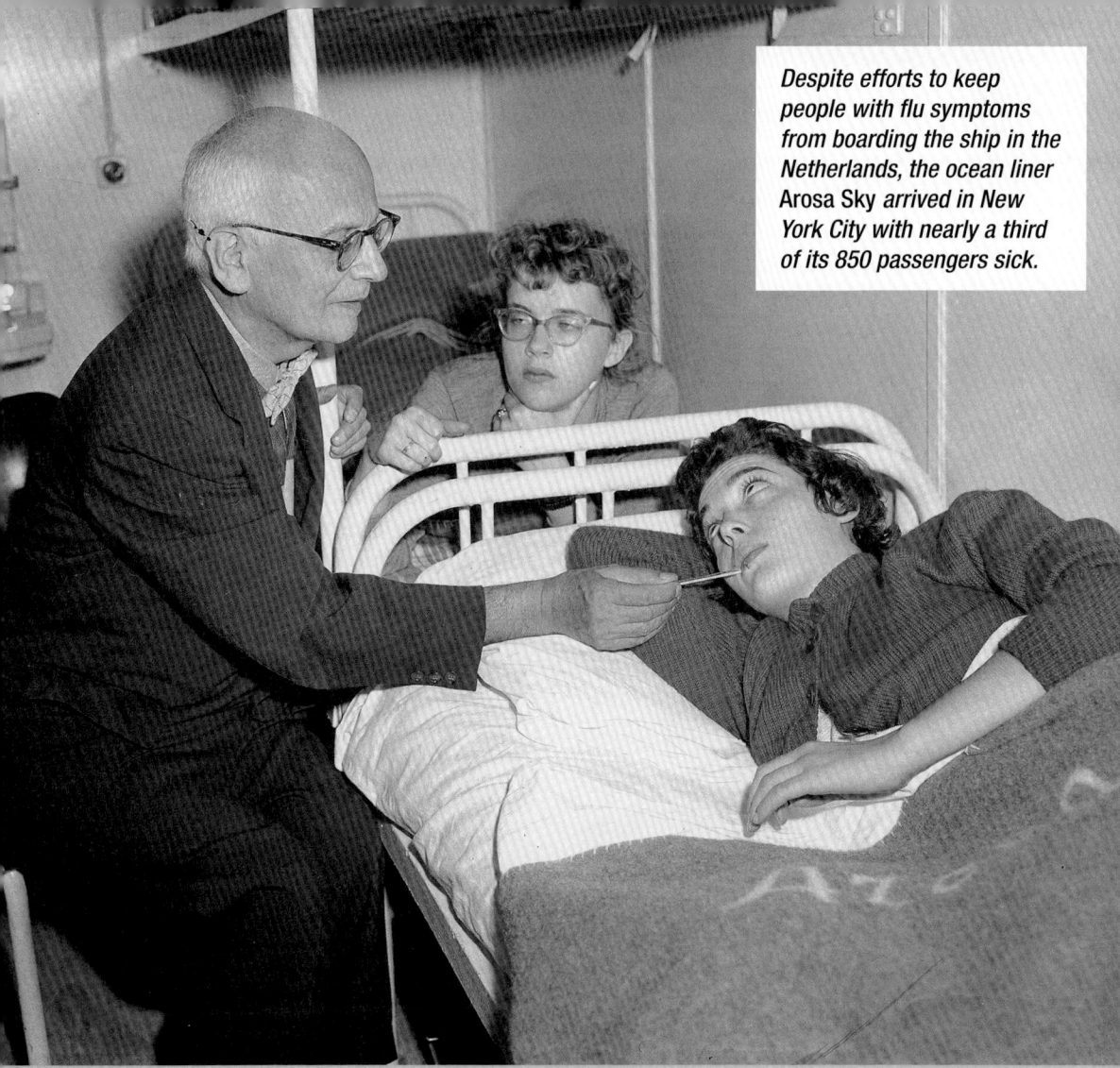

Despite efforts to keep people with flu symptoms from boarding the ship in the Netherlands, the ocean liner *Arosa Sky* arrived in New York City with nearly a third of its 850 passengers sick.

Arosa Sky, which had banned the students, arrived five days later with 250 of its 850 passengers presenting flu symptoms. Even when screening measures were in place, it seems that they were largely ineffective in preventing contagion across borders.

Industrial Absenteeism, Business Closures, and Economic Impacts

As the pandemic spread from country to country, absenteeism affected businesses across the world, but only a few chose to close. In June 1957, for example, motion picture theaters and

School Absenteeism

Absenteeism varied in school districts across the United States during the Asian flu pandemic of 1957. On October 19, 23 percent of students were absent from school in Washington, DC. In nearby Maryland at the same time, comparatively fewer— only 10 percent of students—were recorded absent. Meanwhile, on October 8, New York City's Board of Education had reported that 30 percent of its 965,000 students were absent.

There were repercussions to school funding because of student absenteeism during the pandemic. In New York, for example, the state reduced the amount of money it supplied to New York City public schools in education aid by about two dollars per student for each day of absence. Moreover, the *New York Times* reports that on October 7, 1957, when the pandemic was near its peak, the city lost $560,000 in education funding from the state. New York City's regular loss from absenteeism during that time period was $150,000.

swimming pools were ordered closed in New Delhi, India. Additionally, on November 29, 1957, the *Manchester Guardian* reported that some factories, offices, and mines in the United Kingdom were closed due to the Asian flu. There is no evidence to suggest that these closures limited the spread of the pandemic, particularly in densely populated areas.

The main concern of American businesses at the time of the pandemic was that they were operating on skeletal staffs due to large numbers of employees being at home sick. On October 22, 1957, for example, General Electric reported that there were eighteen hundred employees absent, about 6 percent of its workforce. During the same month, Bell System, a nationwide telephone company, experienced peak industrial absenteeism, with an estimated 8–10 percent of the workforce absent from thirty-six cities. These rates were a bit higher than employee absentee trends across the rest of the country during that time. During the pandemic's peak in October 1957, worker absenteeism in the United States is believed to have ranged anywhere from 3 to 8 percent.

Though there were other factors involved, absenteeism during the pandemic contributed to a recession in the United States, which subsequently spread globally. The economic downturn began at the end of 1957 and continued to May 1958. In the journal *Pathogens*, Patrick R. Saunders-Hastings and Daniel Krewski report that the Asian flu pandemic reduced industrial production by about 1 percent in the United States and by roughly 1.2 percent in Canada.

There were also secondary effects of worker and student absenteeism, like a reduction in transit income in major cities. In densely populated areas, employees and students often used public transportation systems to get to work and school. In October 1957, the New York City Transit Authority reported a $1,185,486 reduction in public transport revenue from the previous month. The *New York Times* reported at the time, "The decrease in the number of passengers—7,984 - 950 in a single month—coincided, the agency reasons, with a fall in school attendance and a rise in industrial absenteeism, including its own."[27] In brief, industries were struggling more because workers were falling ill and being absent rather than because governments were shutting down businesses to contain the spread of the pandemic.

Pandemic Preparedness and Health Information Campaigns

Similarly, pandemic preparedness efforts and health information campaigns tended to focus on treating symptoms and briefing local medical staff more than containing the spread. During the pandemic, there was no government encouragement for citizens to practice social distancing or to refrain from traveling to prevent spread in the United States. Rather, the American Medical Association (AMA) projected that 15–20 percent of the population would contract the virus before a vaccine was available. There was little to no discussion on efforts to reduce that rate of infection.

The Public Health Service seemed to accept contagion as an inevitability and worked with the AMA to ready the country for the pandemic. On July 27, 1957, the AMA set up a committee on influenza to implement a preparedness program. The program involved communicating with doctors about how to handle influenza, making plans at the national level to use all medical personnel, coordinating health departments at the state and local levels, and en-

Health departments used pamphlets, modeled on this one that had been created during the Spanish flu pandemic, to inform the public about how to prevent the spread of influenza.

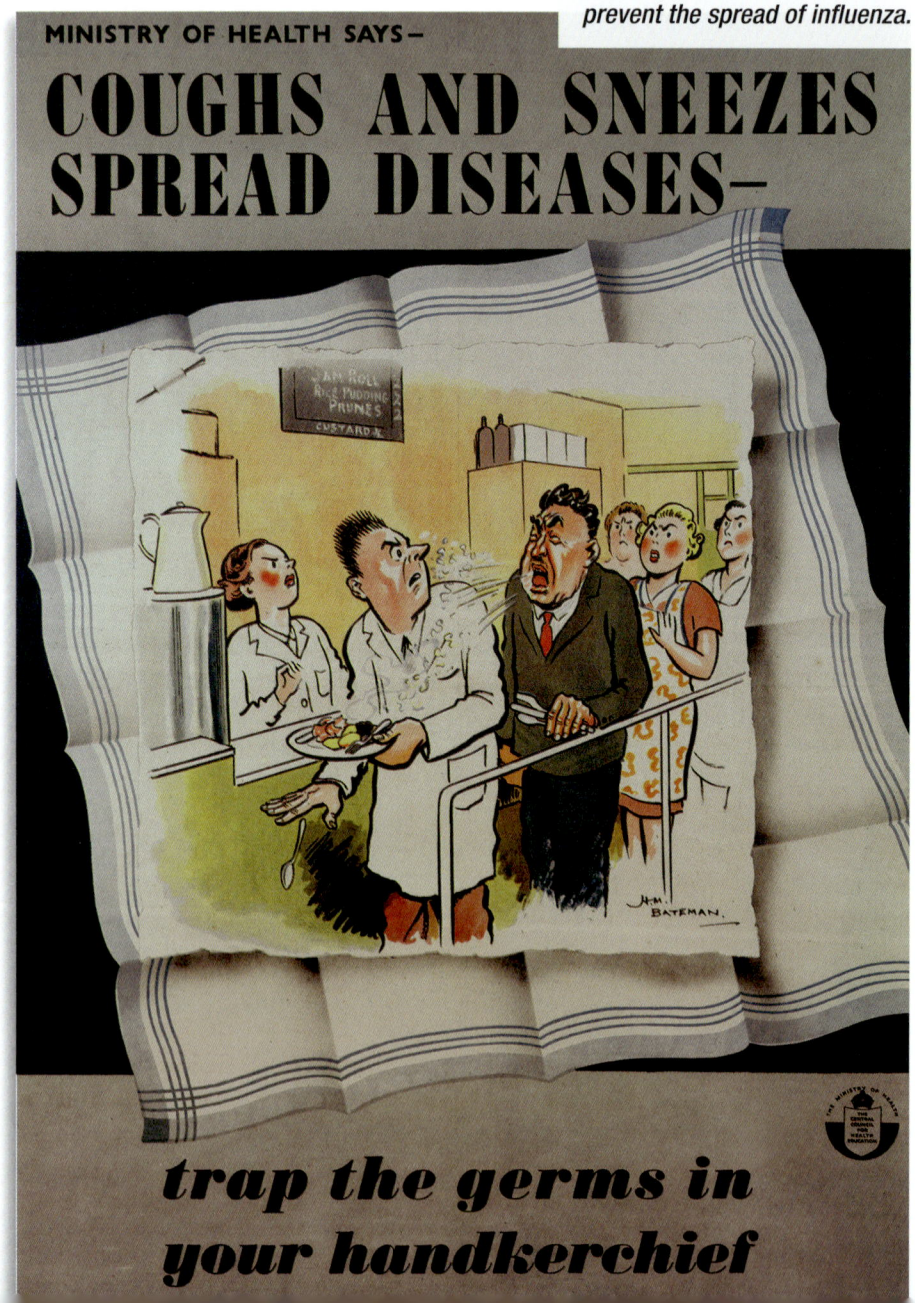

couraging state and local medical societies to make epidemic emergency preparedness plans. During its planning and coordination efforts, the AMA stressed to the public that there was "no immediate cause for alarm."[28] Harold C. Leuth, chairman of the AMA's special committee on influenza, explained the necessity of emergency preparedness and coordination. He said, "Rapid onset of the epidemic makes it mandatory to have plans prepared well in advance and to see that the 1,911 medical societies in the country are cognizant of the magnitude of the problem before the epidemic strikes."[29]

Aside from preparing medical staff, information campaigns were launched to educate the public about how to treat symptoms from the Asian flu. In October 1957, the New York City Health Department, for example, distributed 250,000 pamphlets on what to do if Asian flu were to strike a household. It also made 1 million summaries with the same information, which it offered to libraries, schools, and drugstores in the city. As cases surged, patients requiring medical treatment were offered aspirin, cough medicine, and nose drops, and they were then (with very few exceptions) sent home from the hospital. The distributed pamphlets encouraged those afflicted to treat symptoms like they would for a cold: rest, drink fluids, take aspirin, and stay home from work or school.

Although health information campaigns and the media made the public aware of the Asian flu's symptoms and treatment, public officials worldwide did relatively little to curb the spread of the pandemic. With few exceptions, children continued to attend school, play sports, and socialize with their friends. Adults went to work until they fell ill. And families continued traveling for holidays. Despite the highly contagious nature and slightly increased mortality rate of the new influenza virus, people lived as they had before. In the *Pathogens* article discussing the history of pandemic influenza, Saunders-Hastings and Krewski write, "There was little use of non-pharmaceutical interventions, such as school closure, travel restrictions, banning of mass gatherings, or quarantine. Quarantine, in particular, was considered inappropriate due to the mild nature of symptoms and the large overall number of infections."[30] When small attempts were made to alleviate the spread, like with the limits on public gatherings in Cochise County, Arizona, the public officials' efforts were comparable to plugging one small hole on a sinking ship containing many holes. They might have made a slight difference, but it was virtually unnoticeable.

CHAPTER FOUR

The Determined Pioneer and a Timely Vaccine

In April 1957 Maurice Hilleman, a microbiologist and the chief of the Department of Respiratory Diseases at Walter Reed Army Medical Center, read an article in the *New York Times* picturing Asian flu patients in Hong Kong. *National Geographic* reports that Hilleman said, "My God. This is the pandemic. It's here!"[31] The day after reading the article, Hilleman sent a cable to an army medical general laboratory in Zama, Japan, requesting virus samples.

In May 1957, preceding the pandemic's arrival in the United States, Hilleman received a virus sample (in the form of gargled salt water) from an ill member of the US Navy who had been to Hong Kong. Hilleman sent the incubated virus to other research organizations for assistance. Scientists from these organizations determined that most people did not have the antibody necessary to fight the new virus, with the exception of a few elderly people who had survived the Russian flu pandemic of 1889–1890. This confirmed what Hilleman had suspected: the virus was highly contagious and would course through populations worldwide. He took initiative to call for the production of an Asian flu vaccine and facilitate its distribution to millions of people.

Hilleman's Background

Hilleman's early life and upbringing contributed to his determination to create vaccines. He was born in 1919 during the Spanish influenza pandemic, the deadliest influenza pandemic in history. He was raised on a farm in Montana. In high school, he took a job as an assistant manager at J.C. Penney before his brother convinced him to apply for a college scholarship. After finishing his bachelor's degree at Montana State University, he went on to get his doctorate in microbiology at the University of Chicago. Upon completion in 1944, he began working for a pharmaceutical company developing vaccines. In an interview with Paul Offit, who published a biography of Hilleman titled *Vaccinated: One Man's Quest to Defeat the World's Deadliest Diseases*, Hilleman explained that his decision to work with pharmaceuticals was un-

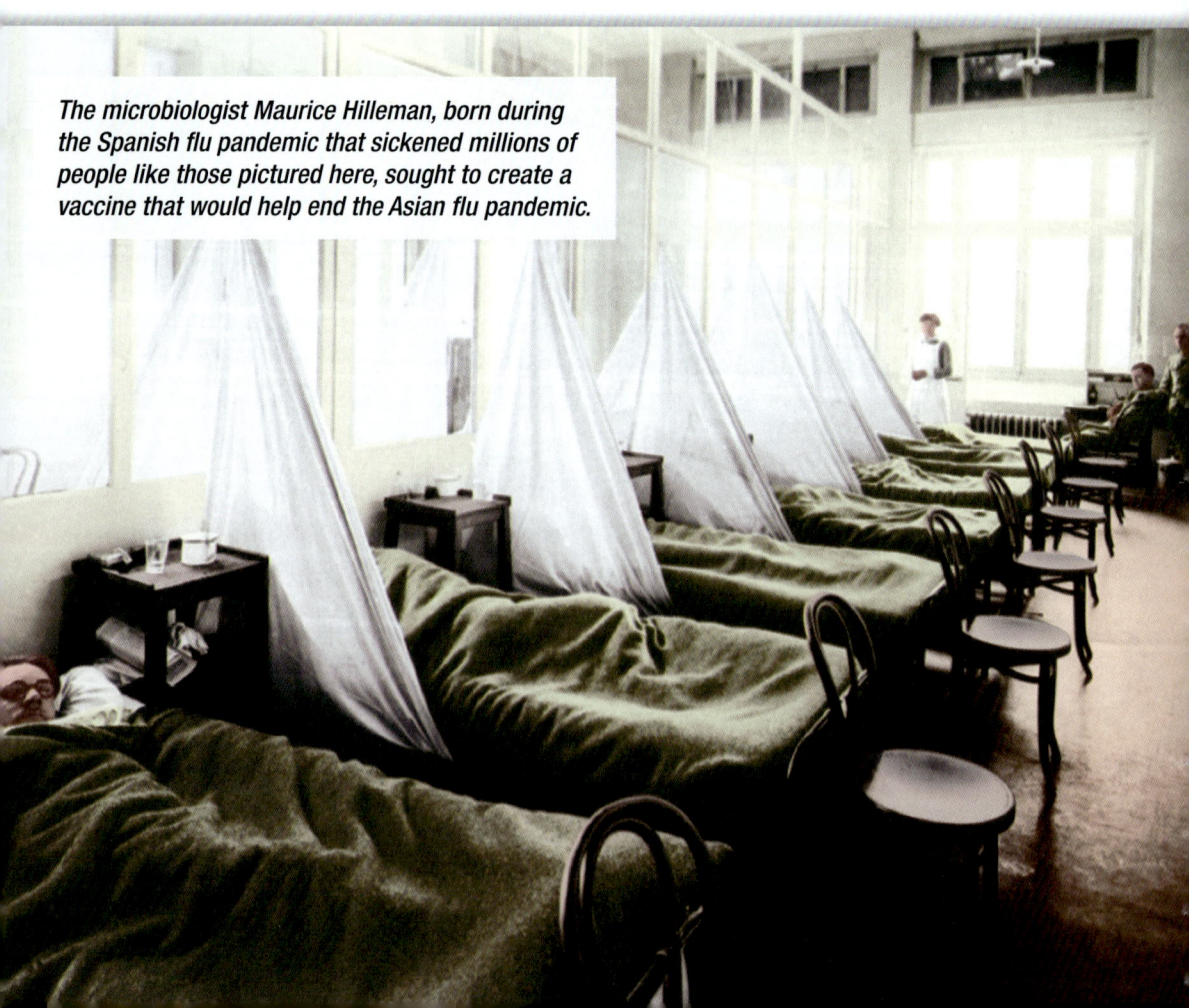

The microbiologist Maurice Hilleman, born during the Spanish flu pandemic that sickened millions of people like those pictured here, sought to create a vaccine that would help end the Asian flu pandemic.

popular among his advisers. Graduates from the University of Chicago, one of the nation's premier educational institutions, were expected to stay in academia and continue researching and teaching. Hilleman, however, wanted to pursue a different type of life. He said, "I came off a farm. We had to do marketing. We had to do sales. I wanted to do something. I wanted to make things!"[32]

After spending four years at E.R. Squibb researching and learning how to mass-produce influenza vaccines, in the spring of 1948 Hilleman took a position at Walter Reed Army Medical Center. According to Offit, Hilleman's job was to "learn everything he could about influenza and to prevent the next pandemic."[33]

The Race Against the Clock

Knowing there was little time to produce a vaccine before the Asian flu reached US shores, Hilleman realized he had to act quickly. He had little success when he first contacted government officials. In Hilleman's biography, Offit reports that Joseph Bell, the assistant surgeon of the US Public Health Service, did not agree with Hilleman on the severity of the impending pandemic. Bell's response to the crisis was, "What pandemic? What influenza?"[34]

The head of the influenza commission for the US military, Thomas Francis, also did not initially believe the world was dealing with another pandemic and was unwilling to work on the vaccine. Hilleman, however, was known among his contemporaries for his determination. He knew that Francis was scheduled to have dinner one night at the Cosmos Club in Washington, DC, so he waited for him there at the door. Hilleman recalls approaching him personally and saying, "Thomas Francis, I've got to show you something because you're making a huge mistake. We don't have time to fool around."[35] Perhaps persuaded in part by Hilleman's persistence, Francis was convinced after having perused the data. He concluded, "My God, it's a pandemic virus."[36]

Though Hilleman convinced some officials, he continued to meet resistance from others. When Hilleman was about to issue a press release suggesting the time frame that the virus would enter the United States—the first week of school in September 1957— some public officials vehemently disagreed. Hilleman recalled, "I was declared crazy. But it came, on time."[37]

Getting little support from the government in his quest, Hilleman worked to organize vaccine production directly with pharmaceutical manufacturers. He reportedly ignored the US principal vaccines, regulatory agency, the Division of Biologics Standards, by calling vaccine manufacturing companies himself. He sent virus samples to the pharmaceutical companies and encouraged them to develop a vaccine in four months. Hilleman recognized that four months was a short timeline, but he requested that manufacturers do as he was doing and bypass the bureaucracy. Hilleman and the vaccine's manufacturers were working on an unprecedented mission. The Asian flu marked the first time that a modern pandemic influenza virus could be investigated in a laboratory. Technological innovations and advancements associated with epidemiology and virology were able to rise to the challenge of potentially defeating a pandemic before it ran its course.

Hilleman further had the foresight to take measures to fortify egg supplies across the United States. Chicken eggs are needed to incubate viruses so that the antigens can be harvested and injected—as part of the vaccine—into humans. The antigens are those parts of the pathogen that trigger an immune response from the body. Because of his experience on the farm in Montana, Hilleman knew well that roosters were normally killed late in the hatching season because they were useless for meat production and they could not lay eggs. Therefore, he requested that the farming community keep roosters alive to fertilize enough eggs for millions of vaccine doses—an estimated hundreds of thousands of eggs a day.

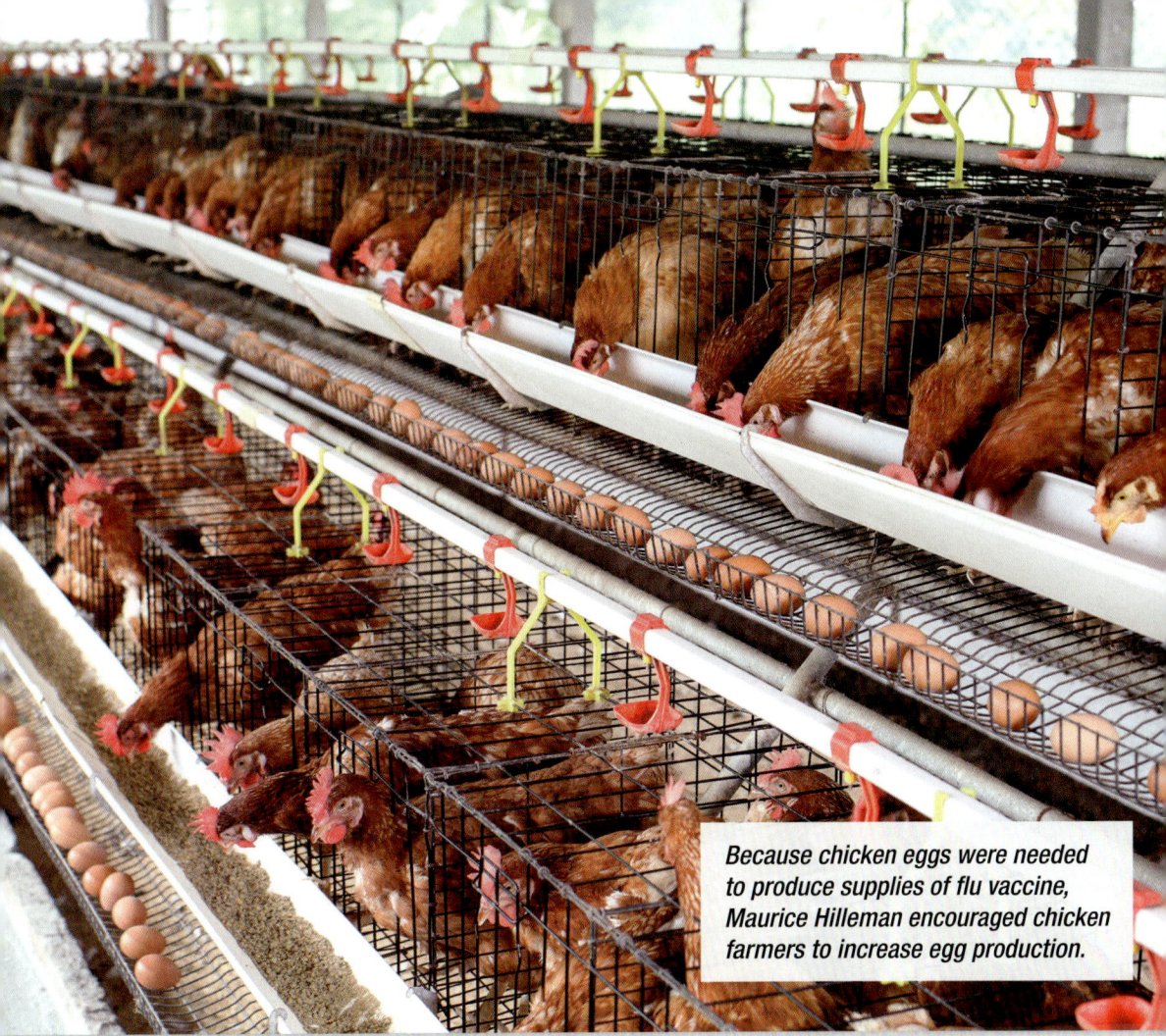

Because chicken eggs were needed to produce supplies of flu vaccine, Maurice Hilleman encouraged chicken farmers to increase egg production.

Funding and Distribution

Hilleman's efforts with the farming community yielded results. His initiative in pushing the government to support a vaccination program also paid off. President Eisenhower, though aware of the Asian flu pandemic early on, was not initially interested in supporting a vaccination program. As Hilleman's perspective gained momentum and the virus reached the United States, public officials seemed to reconsider their lack of support for a vaccine. In August Eisenhower asked Congress for $500,000 in funding for the Public Health Service. He further asked to transfer $2 million in public health funds to fight the pandemic. He set a goal of 60 million vaccines by February 1, 1958, enough to vaccinate a third of the US population.

By the time the president publicly supported the vaccination initiative in August, it was already well on its way. On June 23, 1957, pharmaceutical corporation Merck & Co. announced that it had created a vaccine it could mass-produce. The National Institutes of Health tested the vaccine, which was later estimated to be 60 to 80 percent effective. In July, the vaccinations were administered slowly as they became available. In August Dr. William Stewart, the assistant to the US surgeon general, warned health officers, "People need to know that there is not going to be enough vaccine for everybody for a while, and those who take care of us while we are sick or provide essential community services should get the vaccine first."[38] After health care workers, military personnel, and first responders received their doses, people with chronic illnesses such as heart conditions, diabetes, and tuberculosis were next in line for the vaccine. At the end of August, the American Academy of Pediatrics reported that the vaccine was safe for children over three months old and was to be administered in two doses for children under thirteen years old. By the end of August, over 1 million vaccines had been administered. Three months later, in November, medical professionals had vaccinated 40 million people in the United States.

Leading by Example

President Eisenhower was among those vaccinated. On August 26, 1957, after his repeated refusals, the president got his Asian flu vaccination. When initially given the opportunity to get inoculated, the president said that he wanted to be treated like an average citizen and not get special treatment, but when the Public Health Service recommended that older people with chronic illnesses should be vaccinated first, sixty-six-year-old Eisenhower decided to lead by example and get his shot.

In contrast, Dr. Thomas Ward did not. Ward, an associate professor at the University of Notre Dame's LOBUND Laboratories, was directing tests of the vaccine for the Public Health Service. He declined the vaccine for himself in early September. He said he preferred instead to build his immunity naturally. According to Ward, the seriousness of the virus was exaggerated and was only an issue for children under age three and adults over sixty.

During the time Ward was testing vaccine safety in the United States, other nations were developing vaccines for the Asian flu as well. For example, vaccines in the United Kingdom were produced at the Wright-Fleming Institute of Microbiology in west London and distributed in October 1957. Japanese laboratories had prepared only 1.5 million vaccines by November 1957. In some countries, such as Japan, vaccines were not carried out

Eggs and Vaccines

Eggs are used in many vaccines. Therefore, when people are given certain vaccines, medical professionals ask them if they have an egg allergy. During the 1930s, Ernest Goodpasture, an American pathologist and pioneer of virology, discovered that viruses could be grown in eggs. Thomas Francis, who was the head of the influenza commission for the US military when Hilleman approached him at the Cosmos Club in 1957, was the first to use eggs for an influenza vaccine during the 1940s, when he was conducting research at the University of Michigan. Francis grew the influenza virus in the egg and then killed it with formaldehyde, a simple chemical compound made of hydrogen, oxygen, and carbon. Hilleman used a similar technique for many subsequent vaccines during his lifetime.

The CDC reports that when vaccines are made, the viruses are injected into fertilized eggs and incubated for several days to allow the viruses to replicate. The fluid containing the virus is harvested from the eggs. The virus is then killed and purified. When the inactive virus antigens are injected into its host, the body produces antibodies to protect the recipient against the antigens and thus against a live virus that possesses them.

on a wide scale but were given instead to priority groups. In others, vaccines were not used much at all. Vaccine manufacturers were located in developed countries, making it much less likely that citizens in countries such as Brazil, India, or Nigeria had access to a vaccine. In places where there was not a largely distributed vaccine, transmission of the virus was eventually slowed by herd immunity, in which 60 percent of the population has been infected and the transmission rate slows only because the virus has fewer unprotected hosts to infect.

The Virus Lingers

Relying on herd immunity to end a pandemic is a costly strategy. More vulnerable people contract the virus, so there are inevitably more deaths. The Asian flu pandemic killed between 70,000 and 116,000 people in the United States alone. Public health experts estimate that there would have been 1 million deaths in the United States without the vaccine. Hilleman later reflected on the accomplishment by stating, "That's the only time we ever averted a pandemic with a vaccine."[39]

Even in the places where people had access to the vaccine, the Asian flu still lingered for years, just not at epidemic levels. The pandemic peaked in the United States in October 1957. With the widespread introduction of the vaccine into the population, numbers decreased throughout the autumn and winter of 1957–1958. The US surgeon general announced that new cases had decreased from 1,250,000 in the first week of November to 225,000 in the last week of that month. By December 1957, it seemed that the rush to get the vaccine had passed. On December 8, the *New York Times* reported that as the pandemic subsided, so too did demand for the vaccine. Vaccine producers grew concerned with their investment as laboratories stored large excess inventories of the Asian flu vaccine. Fortunately, the vaccines could be stored for eighteen months under refrigeration, and the manufacturers had extensive contracts to provide doses for the military. Despite the success and availability of a

A Potentially Dangerous Mistake

On April 12, 2005, WHO announced that between October 2004 and February 2005 the College of American Pathologists (CAP) had mistakenly sent samples of the influenza A (H2N2) virus, the culprit for the 1957 pandemic, to 3,747 labs. All but 75 of those labs were in the United States. CAP paid Meridian Bioscience of Cincinnati, a private company, to prepare and send the samples as part of a routine testing program. Labs receive viral samples periodically to test their proficiency at identifying viruses.

Sending this virus by mistake could have proved dangerous. Anyone born after 1968 would have little or no immunity to the H2N2 virus, and the vaccine was no longer available. Therefore, WHO recommended that the samples should be destroyed upon receipt. Klaus Stohr, chief of WHO's global influenza program, called the decision to send Asian flu samples "unwise" and stated, "The risk is relatively low that a lab worker will get sick, but a large number of labs got it and if someone does get infected, the risk of illness is high and this virus has shown to be fully transmissible."

Quoted in Center for Infectious Disease Research and Policy, "Pandemic Flu Virus from 1957 Mistakenly Sent to Labs," University of Minnesota, April 13, 2005. https://www.cidrap.umn.edu.

vaccine in the United States, with a substantial number of hosts remaining in the population and a 70 percent efficacy rate, the virus persisted.

Throughout the winter, cities reported a second wave of the Asian flu. In February 1958, the Public Health Service reported that influenza and pneumonia deaths had increased for the previous four weeks in 108 US cities. On February 11, the *New York Times* reported that Milwaukee, Wisconsin, noted a second wave of the Asian flu that approached an epidemic level.

The following winter, public health experts across the United States downgraded the threat of the Asian flu. For example, on September 23, 1958, New York state health commissioner Herman E. Hilleboe said that there was little likelihood the Asian flu would significantly impact the state. He did recommend, however, that the elderly, pregnant women, and people susceptible to respiratory illnesses should get the flu vaccine.

For many years following Hilleman's Asian flu vaccine quest of 1957, pharmaceutical companies included the Asian flu in their annual multistrain flu vaccines. In 1962, US surgeon general Luther Terry predicted there would be renewed outbreaks of Asian flu across the country. He recommended that everyone over age forty-five—not just those over sixty-five, as was the norm at that time—should get their flu vaccine containing the Asian flu antigens. Terry and other public health officials warned that the Asian flu seemed to occur in cycles of two to three years.

As it turned out, the surgeon general was correct. An Asian flu outbreak in New York City reached epidemic levels in February 1963. Additionally, the Public Health Service's Communicable Disease Center reported Asian flu outbreaks in three counties in Kansas during the same time. The center further reported outbreaks of suspected Asian flu in fifteen states and the District of Columbia. On July 7, 1963, the *New York Times* reported that an additional 11,125 people in the United States had died as a result of the Asian flu that winter.

Defeating a Pandemic

By 1968 the virus had run its course and was extinct in the human population. It was believed to be extinct in the wild as well. Public health experts think that the Asian flu pandemic would have run a much more devastating course in the United States had it not been for Maurice Hilleman. After the Asian flu, Hilleman went on to create forty vaccines. His vaccinations included nine of fourteen vaccines presently recommended for children. The US military awarded Hilleman a Distinguished Service Medal for his work. In 1988 he also received the National Medal of Science for his contributions to public health.

When the Asian flu took the world by storm in 1957, it seems that Maurice Hilleman's background, education, and experience made him the inevitable choice to captain its demise. Hilleman's desire to work in industry, rather than conduct research and teach

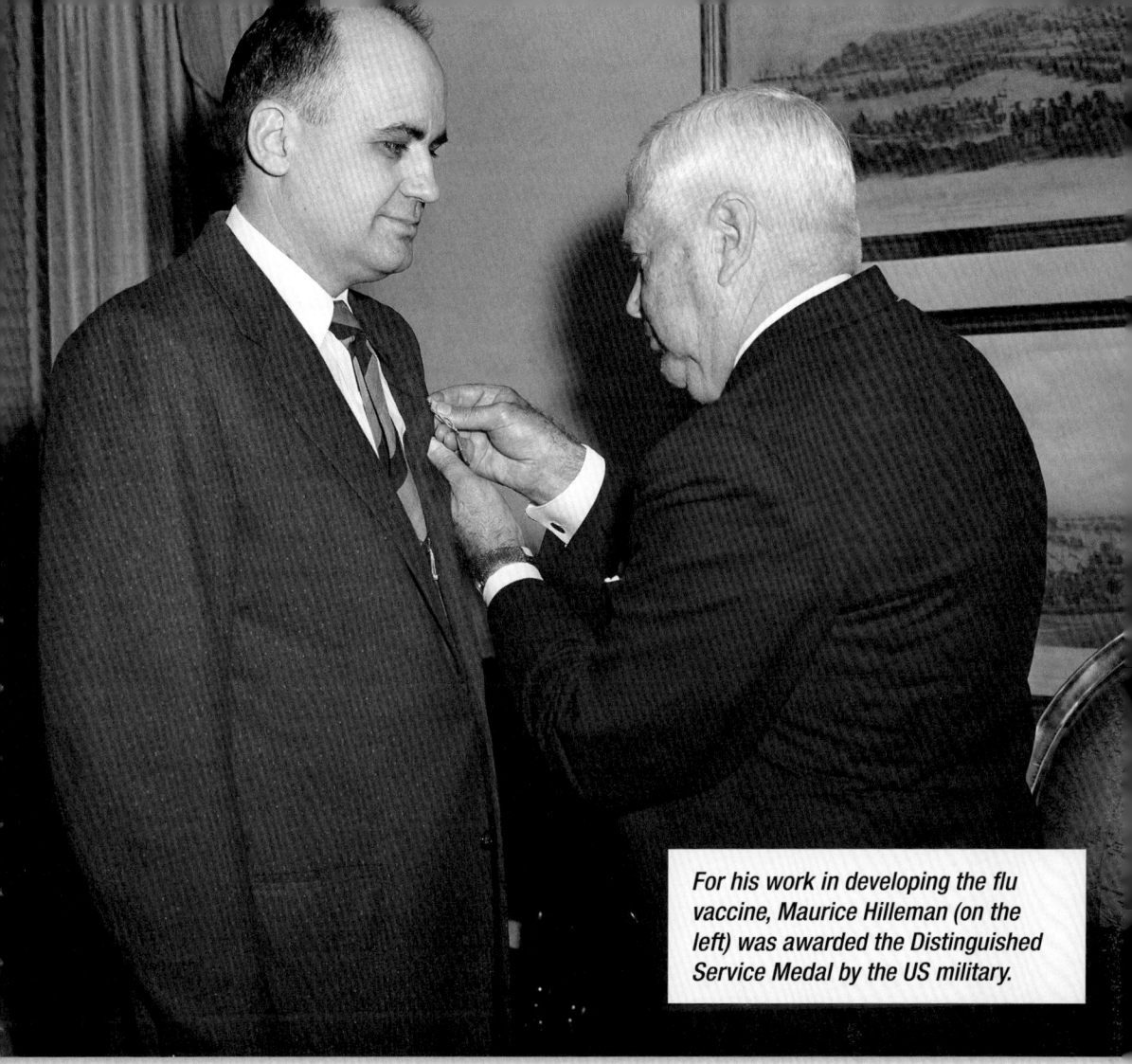

For his work in developing the flu vaccine, Maurice Hilleman (on the left) was awarded the Distinguished Service Medal by the US military.

following his elite graduate education, put him in a position to face the pandemic. His determination and unorthodox approach led him to bypass the regulatory agencies and reach out to vaccine manufacturers himself to get the process started. And the interesting marriage of initiative, scientific innovations, and circumstance led to positive outcomes in defeating the 1957 Asian flu virus.

SOURCE NOTES

Introduction: A Quick Response Saves Lives

1. J. Cavanaugh Simpson, "The Man Who Beat the 1957 Flu Pandemic," *Observations* (blog), *Scientific American*, April 19, 2020. https://blogs.scientificamerican.com.
2. Quoted in Sepp Jannotta, "The Man Who Saved Millions," *Mountains and Minds*, Fall 2012. www.montana.edu.
3. *Life*, "The Asiatic Flu: U.S. Mobilizes to Keep 30 Million People from Succumbing to Epidemic," September 2, 1957, p. 113.

Chapter One: A New Strain of Flu

4. Quoted in John Kelly, "In 1957, a New Flu Appeared in Asia. The World Watched and Waited for It to Spread," *Washington Post*, March 17, 2020. www.washington post.com.
5. *Straits Times*, "Singapore Flu Scare," May 7, 1957. https://eresources.nlb.gov.sg.
6. *New York Times*, "Hong Kong Battling Influenza Epidemic," April 17, 1957. https://timesmachine.nytimes.com.
7. Quoted in *New York Times*, "Influenza Rages in Singapore," May 5, 1957. https://timesmachine.nytimes.com.
8. Sumi Krishna, "I Survived a Pandemic in the Last Century. Now I Fight One More," *The Wire*, March 4, 2020. https://science.thewire.in.
9. Harvey Morris, "Asian Flu v. Coronavirus: A Different Time, Similar Problem," News Decoder, March 5, 2020. https://news-decoder.com.
10. Krishna, "I Survived a Pandemic in the Last Century."
11. *New York Times*, "Beniamino Gigli, Famed Tenor, Dies," December 1, 1957. https://timesmachine.nytimes.com.
12. Clark Whelton, "Say Your Prayers and Take Your Chances: Remembering the 1957 Asian Flu Pandemic," *City Journal*, March 19, 2020. www.city-journal.org.

13. Quoted in George P. Larrick, "The FDA Reports to the NARD," *Food, Drug, Cosmetic Law Journal*, November 1957, vol. 12, no. 11, p. 681.

Chapter Two: The Rise of the Pandemic
14. Quoted in Kavita Sivaramakrishnan, "Endemic Risks: Influenza Pandemics, Public Health, and Making Self-Reliant Indian Citizens," *Journal of Global History*, 2020, vol. 15, no. 3, pp. 459–77.
15. Quoted in John Kelly, "Remembering the Asian Flu," *Washington Post*, March 24, 2020. www.washingtonpost.com.
16. Quoted in *Daily Iowan*, "Flu Epidemic Hits Grinnell Assembly," July 2, 1957, p. 6. http://dailyiowan.lib.uiowa.edu.
17. Quoted in Kelly, "In 1957, a New Flu Appeared in Asia."
18. Quoted in Claire Jackson, "History Lessons: The Asian Flu Pandemic," *British Journal of General Practice*, August 1, 2009, vol. 59, pp. 622–23. www.ncbi.nlm.nih.gov.
19. Quoted in *Manchester Guardian*, "Too Much Alarm over Asian Flu," August 30, 1957, p. 14.
20. Quoted in Claire Jackson, "History Lessons."

Chapter Three: Containing the Spread
21. Quoted in John Kelly, "When Flu Cut Mount Holyoke Off from the World in 1957, the Men of Yale Dropped In," *Washington Post*, March 23, 2020. www.washingtonpost.com.
22. Quoted in Kelly, "When Flu Cut Mount Holyoke Off from the World in 1957, the Men of Yale Dropped In."
23. Quoted in Jeff Wilkin, "Asian Flu 1957: How the Region Coped with Another Pandemic," *Daily Gazette*, March 15, 2020. https://dailygazette.com.
24. Quoted in Wilkin, "Asian Flu 1957."
25. *Public Health Reports*, "Health Officers' Meeting on Asian Influenza," November 1957, vol. 72, no. 11, pp. 998–1000. www.ncbi.nlm.nih.gov.
26. Quoted in Bess Furman, "U.S. Acts to Bar Asian Influenza," *New York Times*, June 8, 1957, pp. 21–22. https://timesmachine.nytimes.com.
27. Stanley Levey, "Flu Costs Million in Transit Income," *New York Times*, November 13, 1957, p. 37. https://timesmachine.nytimes.com.

28. Quoted in *New York Times*, "U.S. Put on Alert for Asiatic Flu," July 28, 1957. https://timesmachine.nytimes.com.
29. Quoted in *New York Times*, "U.S. Put on Alert for Asiatic Flu."
30. Patrick R. Saunders-Hastings and Daniel Krewski, "Reviewing the History of Pandemic Influenza: Understanding Patterns of Emergence and Transmission," *Pathogens*, December 2016, vol. 5, no. 4. www.ncbi.nlm.nih.gov.

Chapter Four: The Determined Pioneer and a Timely Vaccine

31. Quoted in Sydney Combs, "The Virologist Saved Millions of Children—and Stopped a Pandemic," *National Geographic*, May 29, 2020. www.nationalgeographic.com.
32. Quoted in Paul Offit, *Vaccinated: One Man's Quest to Defeat the World's Deadliest Diseases*. New York: HarperCollins, 2007, p. 11.
33. Offit, *Vaccinated*, p. 11.
34. Quoted in Offit, *Vaccinated,* p. 14.
35. Quoted in Offit, *Vaccinated*, p. 15.
36. Quoted in Offit, *Vaccinated*, p. 15.
37. Quoted in Offit, *Vaccinated*, p. 15.
38. Quoted in *New York Times*, "More Flu Vaccine Made Available," August 28, 1957, p. 29. https://timesmachine.nytimes.com.
39. Quoted in Combs, "The Virologist Saved Millions of Children."

FOR FURTHER RESEARCH

Books

Don Nardo, *COVID-19 and Other Pandemics: A Comparison*. San Diego: ReferencePoint, 2021.

Paul Offit, *Vaccinated: One Man's Quest to Defeat the World's Deadliest Diseases*. New York: HarperCollins, 2007.

Heather E. Quinlan, *Plagues, Pandemics and Viruses: From the Plague of Athens to COVID 19*. Canton, MI: Visible Ink, 2020.

Internet Sources

Mark Honigsbaum, "Revisiting the 1957 and 1968 Influenza Pandemics," *Lancet*, June 13, 2020. www.thelancet.com.

John Kelly, "In 1957, a New Flu Appeared in Asia. The World Watched and Waited for It to Spread," *Washington Post*, March 17, 2020. www.washingtonpost.com.

Harvey Morris, "Asian Flu v. Coronavirus: A Different Time, Similar Problem," News Decoder, March 5, 2020. https://news-decoder.com.

New York Times, "Hong Kong Battling Influenza Epidemic," April 17, 1957, p. 3. https://timesmachine.nytimes.com.

Paul A. Offit, "The Philly Vaccine Pioneer Who Saved Thousands from Flu, and Predicted the Next Pandemic," *Philadelphia Inquirer*, January 25, 2018. https://www.inquirer.com.

Patrick R. Saunders-Hastings and Daniel Krewski, "Reviewing the History of Pandemic Influenza: Understanding Patterns of Emergence and Transmission," *Pathogens*, December 2016, vol. 5, no. 4. www.ncbi.nlm.nih.gov.

Clark Whelton, "Say Your Prayers and Take Your Chances: Remembering the 1957 Asian Flu Pandemic," *City Journal*, March 13, 2020. https://www.city-journal.org.

PICTURE CREDITS